Healthy Body

First published by Busybird Publishing 2017

ISBN
Print: 978-1-925585-57-5
Ebook: 978-1-925585-58-2

Cover image: Kev Howlett, Busybird Publishing
Cover design: Busybird Publishing
Layout and typesetting: Busybird Publishing

Busybird Publishing
2/118 Para Road
Montmorency, Victoria
Australia 3094
www.busybird.com.au

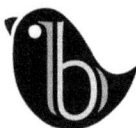

For every book sold, $1 will be donated to the Go for Gold
Scholarship.

'I believe that the greatest gift you can give your family and the world is a healthy you.'

– Joyce Meyer

Contents

Foreword

Carol Cooke AM

'My body is my temple.'

U nfortunately, we are living in a world where people are abusing their temples on a daily basis.

As an elite athlete for most of my life I have tried to take care of my body. This doesn't mean that I have always done the right thing. I've gone through times where I really have let myself down. But after being diagnosed with Multiple Sclerosis in 1998 and wanting to defy the predictions of a very uncaring neurologist, I realised that I needed to really look after my body.

We never understand how much taking care of our bodies can mean until we lose the ability to use it.

In 2001 I was in a wheelchair full time and it was then that I decided to take charge and change the way I was living. It was important for me to look at what I put into my body and make sure that I was doing enough exercise to keep it working the best it could. I did have a bit of medical intervention but I also got back into the water to exercise where I could do things that I couldn't do on land. There was the real possibility that MS would steal my ability to do the things that I loved to do and I didn't want to give those things up. I have been able to defy the predictions of that doctor and go on to win 3 gold medals over 2 Paralympic games and become a five-time world champion in the sport of cycling by taking care of my body and mind.

For without taking care of my body, the mind will not follow.

Our bodies are amazing vessels that, if treated right, will give life, love and happiness for years. Our bodies really do take a pounding throughout our years of living, sometimes not of our own doing. With pollution on the rise and the use of additives to our foods, at times we can be forgiven for not knowing what to do.

This book has some fabulous ideas and suggestions for helping you learn to treat your body as the temple it was meant to be. This isn't a new way of living – we have been thinking about our bodies and health for a long time.

Thales of Miletus – a pre-Socratic Greek philosopher in 546BC – said:

'What man is happy? He who has a healthy body, a resourceful mind, and a docile nature.'

None of us have all the answers, but this book will help you take those first steps to a healthier, better you.

Drink Beer, Be Healthy

Deborah Harrison

This chapter is not about the magical healing or health powers that beer supplies, or about how beer will make you super slim or super fit. This chapter will teach you that you don't need to give up pleasures in life when it comes to food and drink, that you can enjoy them and still stay healthy and happy.

So why call this chapter, 'Drink Beer, Be Healthy'?

For several reasons:

- I personally enjoy a great craft beer.
- My husband is a Head Brewer. That's right! He makes beer for a living.
- I am very passionate about preventing ill-health and chronic disease. The name of my program encouraged men, in particular, to be drawn to our programs for a lifestyle change.
- Beer always gets a bad rap in relation to health. There are a lot of different reasons why we put on weight, and removing one thing – especially one thing that we may love – is not going to work, and certainly not in the long term.

Now, in all honesty, the name of this chapter could have been 'Eat Chocolate, Be Healthy', or, 'Drink Wine, Be Healthy', or whatever your indulgence may be. The important thing is knowing how we can enjoy the things we love and still live a healthy, active life.

The first thing you need to do to change your life is to think about what it is that you want in the future. How much do you value your health, happiness and vitality? Do you want to travel? Climb the Eiffel Tower, visit the pyramids, go on an African Safari, or maybe just buy a caravan and travel around Australia? Do you want to spend more quality time with the grandchildren? To chase them around the park and be an active part of their lives? Do you want to live independently in your own home with a good quality of life with the ones you love?

More importantly, do you want to reduce your risk of developing a range or chronic diseases such as heart disease, type 2 diabetes or cancer?

With age comes life experience, which forms habits and patterns. We have mental, physical, emotional and spiritual needs that need to be met, but finding that balance is often hard to do with all that life throws at us.

This is why looking after our health and wellbeing – through eating nutritionally balanced food, and keeping physically active – is a *must*.

Understanding 'why you do what you do', is the key to creating new patterns, habits, and sustainable changes – especially when your health is at the heart of it all!

Ask yourself:

- Are you an emotional eater?
- Do you eat when you're bored, tired, stressed or sad?
- How much food do you eat in a day?
- What size are your portions of food on your plate?
- What time do you eat your dinner? Is it within 3 hours of going to bed?
- Do you eat out a lot for work or socially?
- Are you constantly surrounded by temptations at work or home?

So many factors contribute to all the good and bad habits you have, but the good news is creating new habits around lifestyle changes are possible with the right support, guidance, motivation, educational tools and knowledge.

As a Nutritionist, Personal Trainer, pilates Instructor and Diabetes Australia educator, you probably assume that when it comes to food and exercise I never step outside the healthy living circle. Truth be told, I still enjoy chocolate, and a glass of beer or wine. My husband and I still go out and enjoy a good meal – although not as often now we have a three-year old – but we still indulge in life's little pleasures.

I understand it is not generally one thing by itself that is the cause of someone being unhealthy. For most people there is going to be more than one part of their life that contributes to their current situation.

There are two main factors that contribute to weight gain or being unhealthy:

1. The first is the types and amount of food we eat.
2. The second is a lack of physical activity.

You cannot get fitter and healthier unless you change both parts of your life. I enjoy dining out, drinking wine and eating chocolate as my rewards, but the rest of the time I eat a healthy, balanced and nutritional diet, drink plenty of water to make sure I keep up my fluid intake, and exercise regularly. I call this my 80/20 rule. Eighty percent of the time I eat well and exercise so I can indulge twenty percent of the time.

The idea of eating healthy is not that hard. It is not counting the calories in food, it is not weighing out food, and it is not ringing up or ordering pre-prepared meals to be sent to your home. In its simplest form, it is about eating a wide variety of nutritious foods from all five food groups and eating them in the right portions. If it does sound easy, that's because it is. All you need to do is to have the right combination of foods when you eat and know which foods are doing what to your body.

Education and knowledge is the key. If you understand how foods impact your health then you can make educated choices on what you decide to put into your body.

Eat plenty of vegetables, legumes and fruits; cereals including breads, rice, pasta, preferably whole grains; include dairy such as milk, yoghurts, cheeses and/or alternatives (preferably reduced fat options); include lean meats, poultry, fish and/or alternatives; and last but not least, drink plenty of water.

Protein

Protein is essential to human life. Your skin, bones, muscles and organ tissue all contain protein. It is also in your blood, hormones and enzymes. Protein is found in many plant foods, as well as many animal sources. Legumes, poultry, seafood, meat, dairy products, nuts and seeds are the richest sources of protein. This is why after a weight workout it's important to replenish your body with protein to help it rebuild and repair the muscles that you have stressed while working out.

Carbohydrates

These are your body's main energy source. Complex carbohydrates include legumes, grains and starchy vegetables such as potatoes, peas and corn.

Simple carbohydrates – also called sugars – are found mainly in fruits and as well as in foods made with sugar as sweets, which basically include most processed and packaged foods.

Complex carbohydrates take longer to breakdown in the body so, as far as sustaining energy, these are the best choices.

Limit your consumption of simple carbohydrates – especially packaged foods. They break down in the body very readily and tend to give you bursts of energy and then are gone, making you want more.

Try not to overeat carbohydrates at night as you are less likely to burn off the calories while you are in your least active state. If your body doesn't use the carbohydrates it will be stored as fat – this is not what you want.

Although carbohydrates are important for fuel, take care not to overindulge, as you need to make sure you'll be able to burn off the fuel.

Fibre

When it comes to a healthy digestive system, most people don't understand the importance of fibre. Fibre is the part of the plant that your body doesn't digest and absorb. There are two basic types: soluble and insoluble. Insoluble fibre adds bulk to your stools and can help prevent constipation. Skins of fruits and vegetables, wheat bran and other whole grains are good sources of insoluble fibre. Soluble fibre may help improve your cholesterol and blood sugar levels. Oats, dried beans, nuts, seeds and some fruits such as apples and oranges are good sources of soluble fibre.

Fats/Oils

The body does require some fats, but not too much, and they need to be the right kind of fats. Fat helps your body absorb many essential vitamins, maintain the structure and function of cell membranes, and preserve the integrity of your immune system. The thing to remember is that fat is a very concentrated energy source, providing twice as many calories per gram as carbohydrates and protein. Too much of certain types of fat – such as saturated fat and trans fat – can increase your blood cholesterol levels and your risk of heart disease. Saturated fats are most often found in animal products such as red meat, poultry, butter and whole milk. Other foods high in saturated fat include coconut, palm and other tropical oils. Saturated fat is the main dietary culprit in raising your blood cholesterol and increasing your risk of heart disease.

Importance of Breakfast

Food is fuel and energy for our bodies and without it we spend the day stumbling around and fighting off a headache. Breakfast is literally just that – breaking the fast that your body was in from the night before. A good breakfast fuels you up and gets you ready for the day.

The consumption of an early morning snack increases the metabolic rate (how fast you burn calories) and kick-starts your body into gear, telling it what to expect for the rest of the day. If breakfast is skipped, your body doesn't process your next meal as quickly, then it tries to hold onto those nutrients as long as possible, instead of burning it right away.

I mentioned earlier about chronic diseases being closely linked to poor health and lack of physical activity. One of the fastest growing lifestyle diseases is type 2 diabetes – so what is it?

Type 2 Diabetes

Type 2 diabetes is often referred to as the 'Lifestyle Disease'. The factors that can put you at high risk are: high blood pressure, being overweight, little or no physical activity and poor diet.

Consuming more food than your body needs to function causes your blood sugar levels to be too high. When your body breaks down the food you eat it turns it into a simple blood sugar called glucose. A steady balance of glucose (blood sugar) and insulin (a hormone released from the pancreas) is needed to maintain normal blood sugar levels.

With type 2 diabetes, your body's cells do not use insulin properly. This results in glucose entering cells which become impaired, called 'insulin resistance'. However, it is a disease that can be easily prevented.

Research shows that although there are different forms of diabetes, type 2 diabetes accounts for 85–90 percent of all diabetes problems currently in Australia. Statistics also show that this is one of the fastest growing chronic diseases, closely linked to Australians also developing heart disease and strokes.

There is a solution! Applying very simple and small lifestyle changes, through the right education on what, when and how you eat, along with regular physical activity, are the keys to preventing this 'lifestyle' disease. The choice is yours.

Finding Time to Relax for Health

Along with eating a well-balanced diet and doing regular physical activity, a healthy lifestyle must also include time to relax and wind down.

Why? Stresses are present every day of our lives and can affect us in many ways. A small amount of stress is not thought to be a bad thing. We all have in-built coping mechanisms which should be activated from time to time, but they are not designed to run continuously. This is where stress-related symptoms start to appear – such as headaches, high blood pressure and heart disease. By taking time out to relax – reading a good book, listening to music, meditating, going for a walk, or taking a yoga, pilates or tai chi class – you can help your body and mind remain healthy.

Worrying about things that happened yesterday or even what may happen tomorrow, next week or next year, is not good for your health or happiness.

One of my favourite quotes puts life into perspective for me:

'Yesterday is history. Tomorrow is a mystery. Today is a gift. That is why is it called the present.'

'Muscle Mass Dictates Metabolism' a Scientific-Based Fact – Exercise and You

My background is also in fitness, and throughout this chapter I have emphasised the importance of regular physical activity along with eating well. Allow me to explain some of its many benefits for optimum health.

As we get older, our bodies build muscle less efficiently, and the muscle we already have breaks down faster. This makes regular exercise an integral part of healthy aging. Many studies over the years have proven that exercise not only helps us maintain our muscle mass, but can also increase it. It keeps our metabolism high, and gives us strength and endurance to complete everyday tasks.

Fitness for men and women – especially load-bearing exercises such as weights, resistance bands and stair climbing – is very important for bone health. These types of exercises can help prevent osteoporosis and maintain bone mass, and even help protect you from falls, which can be a life-changing event as we get older.

We have been hearing for years that regular activity boosts your mood, but it does much more than that. Exercise can make a big difference, and working out can definitely help you relax and improve your mood. When you exercise, neurotransmitters and endorphins that ease stress, worry and anxiety are released. This has been shown to calm nerves and encourage an overall feeling of wellness. Once you get motivated, make it a new habit!

Another benefit of regular exercise that spurs me on to keep going is the fact that exercise can enhance your mental clarity, performance and work productivity. As a mum and successful businesswoman, these things are more important than ever to me.

Pain vs Pleasure Concept

We can all make excuses for not looking after ourselves. I bet somewhere along the line you've moaned and groaned about always being tired, sick and without sufficient time to make your health a real priority.

I like to call this our **'Pain'** factor. It's funny that we would rather stay in this mode of thinking, instead of stepping outside our comfort zone a little. By doing so we would gain so many benefits of increased health and wellbeing, and enjoy living life to the full – what I call our **'Pleasure'** factor.

So how do we push past that pain to receive and enjoy the pleasures of life?

You must identify your personal reasons (your 'why') for wanting to change.

What does being healthy mean to you, your family, and your future? What does it mean in regards to your quality of life? Writing these things down is a great place to start. You could even write down what you think your life will look like in ten years if you choose not to make any changes regarding your health and wellbeing. This can often help to put life in perspective.

My own reasons why I continue to eat and live well relate to my personal family history of heart disease and diabetes. In addition, being a great role model for my family, friends and clients is very important to me. I know I can make a difference to my quality of life with exercise, diet and lifestyle modifications, and hope to inspire them to do the same.

Listed below are more scientifically proven facts that can help to improve, prevent, manage or even eliminate a condition, by adopting simple and small changes to your exercise and eating habits. I am sure one or more of these will resonate with you.

- Increase energy levels
- Reduce stress
- Improve sleep
- Reduced inflammation of the joints
- Decrease cholesterol
- Decrease blood pressure
- Prevent/reduce the risk of developing chronic diseases such as heart disease, type 2 diabetes and strokes
- Reduce and/or eliminate the taking of some medications
- Improve quality of life
- Improve and help manage chronic illnesses
- Increase bone density
- Increase muscle mass (which in turn dictates metabolism)
- Is it time that you made the change for better health and wellbeing?

Deb's 5 Easy Tips for Achieving a Healthier Lifestyle

1. Enjoy five serves (minimum of three cups) of vegetables per day as they help to keep you feeling full for longer, help the digestive system and help prevent certain types of cancers. Lots of green leafy vegetables preferably, the more colours the better, and seasonal variety.

2. Starchy carbohydrates should be kept to a minimum, with one to two small serves per day. These include cereals, bread, rice, pasta. Where possible choose wholegrain varieties.

3. Enjoy at least eight glasses or two litres of water per day. Reduce caffeinated beverages to one to two per day and minimise alcohol intake.

4. Keeping and maintaining a perfect diet 100% of the time can be a challenge. Remember my suggestion with the 80/20 rule – eat well most of the time and enjoy the treats like going out for a great meal paired with a few good beers, wines and even dessert occasionally. This will keep your lifelong wellbeing journey achievable, realistic, enjoyable and sustainable.

5. Aim for 30 minutes of light to moderate exercise most days of the week. Great for stress release as it conditions the body and mind, and encourages the release of the 'happy hormone' called endorphins, which help you feel good. Important to the support of not only the physical but the mental wellbeing.

Prevention is the Key

Think about your health and please put yourself first. Look after you! Look after you so you can live life to the fullest and enjoy and share it with friends, family and loved ones, doing all those things that living a healthy lifestyle can bring. Remember that small changes can be achieved and sustained for life, giving you a healthy future with **quality** of life. Not only empowering you, but those around you too.

> *'If, at the age of 30 you are stiff and out of shape, you are old. If at 60, you are supple and strong, then you are young.'*
> **– Joseph Pilates**

Be inspired!

References

Dietary Guidelines for Australian Adults – Australian Government Department of Health and Ageing
An Active Way to Better Health – Australian Government Department of Health and Ageing
Diabetes Australia Website

Movement is Magic

Nikki Ellis

There are thousands of exercise scientists around the world who have made it their life's work to research how we should best exercise to maintain optimal health. The American College of Sports Medicine (ACSM) is the largest sports medicine and exercise science organisation in the world. It is dedicated to collating, advancing and integrating that research to ensure that exercise professionals like me, as well as the general public, know exactly what we should do to create and maintain a healthy body through exercise.

So, because of this, my job as a personal trainer and educator is easy, right? I can simply let my clients know how they need to be exercising – and they do it!

Well, no. In Australia, we simply are not exercising enough – even though we know we should be doing more. In 2011/12 according to research by the Heart Foundation, over a quarter of males in Australia aged 15 and over had low levels of physical activity, representing 2.5 million male Australians. Over a third of females in Australia aged 15 and over had low levels of exercise, representing 3.1 million female Australians. Like sedentary behaviour, the prevalence of low levels of exercise increases with age. Comparing from 1995 there has been a gradual trend upwards for Australian men and women to have sedentary lifestyles. For many of us, jobs where we sit in front of a computer for long hours, drive home and then sit in front of a television for long hours are creating a shift from the typical Australian being portrayed as the lean bronzed life saver, to one where the typical Aussie is unfit, overweight and sedentary. Have we really become "Norm" from the iconic *Life, Be In It!* Government campaign of the 70s?

So, let's start really simply. With help from the ACSM guidelines, what exactly should we be doing in terms of exercise, to not only stay in shape, but stay free of disease, and feeling full of vigour?

There are four basic elements of exercise that are recommended, and we'll look at each one in turn: cardiorespiratory exercise, resistance exercise, flexibility, and neuro-motor exercise.

Cardiorespiratory Exercise (CV exercise)

Great for heart health and keeping our metabolic rates high, cardio respiratory is the 'huff and puff' training.

Adults should get at least 150 minutes of moderate intensity CV exercise each week. For example, a thirty minute walk five days per week. However, if you prefer to do some vigorous exercise you could do three lots of vigorous exercise for 20–60 mins instead (e.g. three spin classes). Remember that these are guidelines for the minimum amounts – it's quite OK if you want to walk every day and also do some high intensity training as well. Although it is certainly possible to do too much exercise – for most of us this is not an issue. Just ensure you build up slowly.

You can also choose to do your cardio exercise in multiple shorter sessions rather than one continuous session. This is, again, useful when building up fitness. If a 30-minute walk is just too long fitness-wise, or maybe time-wise, going out for three separate walks of at least ten minutes is AOK. (We also know that when people go out for a ten-minute walk they naturally tend to walk for longer than ten minutes anyway – winning!).

Gradually increase both your frequency and your intensity for best adherence to exercise and less risk of injury.

Even if you are not quite able to achieve these minimums, something is always better than nothing! Simply start with what you can do, and build up.

Resistance Exercise

You might tend to call this training 'weight training' but exercise experts prefer resistance training as it doesn't always involve lifting weights. Resistance training encompasses body weight training such as body weight squats, chin-ups or pushups, foam dumbells used in water, Swiss balls, some yoga positions and pilates reformer machines – so, resistance training is a more collective term.

This is an area I am extremely passionate about. I taught resistance training to exercise science students at Victoria University for ten years and feel that this is one area that many people really neglect. Most of us know that we need to walk, but many folks I talk to – especially when I present to older adults at PROBUS clubs – don't realise that resistance training is a key component in maintaining physical health.

Unfortunately, there is still the perception that lifting weights is:

- purely for aesthetics
- just for younger people (especially young men).

In fact, the people who could benefit most from resistance training are older adults.

Resistance training is the BEST activity for bone strength.

Resistance training helps to maintain and increase our muscle size (dependant on training variables, diet and hormonal status), strength and power – which we naturally lose as we age.

Resistance training is excellent at regulating our blood sugar levels – great news for people with diabetes or pre-diabetes.

Resistance training helps to increase feelings of self-worth, self-esteem and self-efficacy – so important, especially in our young adults.

Resistance training helps to improve balance and postural integrity.

Until 2011, resistance training was not included in the American College of Sports Medicine Guidelines as essential exercise – which may be a key reason why so many of us don't think it is 'for us'. The recommendations are that adults should train each major muscle group (legs, back, chest, shoulders) two to three days per week using a variety of equipment.

Start off – especially as an older or sedentary

person – with a light intensity and progress to higher intensity. Even better, train with an experienced personal trainer or exercise physiologist who can gauge your weights for you, develop a well-structured program, and watch your technique.

In terms of sets and reps, starting off at 2–3 sets of 8–15 reps will give you some strength and hypertrophy. Higher reps of 15 or more will increase muscular endurance.

This is all very standard fare – it is safe and practical. Let's presume you are in good health and have a doctor's clearance to train. Start to push yourself a little harder. Just like in our work lives where hard work gets you ahead, so it is with weight training. One of the key mistakes I see in public gyms is patrons coasting along. The younger adults play with their phones for five minutes in between sets, the older adults tend to operate at an effort level a little lower than they should be because they have been told to 'go light' and be ultra-cautious. Whist I absolutely concur that we start slowly and build from there, don't be frightened of making your body work. By the 12th rep or so, you should be struggling to do any more. If you could keep going and do another ten reps, trust me, the load is too light for you. Older adults have been found to be quite OK with coping with challenging loads. Again, I stress I don't mean to go super heavy on your first workout, but once you have a base level of strength (e.g. have been training several months) then start upping the ante.

Flexibility

Recommendations are that adults should do some flexibility training three days a week to improve range of motion. Ideally, we all want to have 'normal' range of motion at all our joints. We don't necessarily need to be super flexible – just normal range is fine. The best time to stretch is immediately post training when muscles and connective tissues are warm and therefore more pliable. Do remember that stretching after you train does not make you less sore (a common misconception). Likewise, doing static stretches BEFORE you train is not a good idea – in fact, it decreases the strength and power of the muscles you are about to use for your lifts – stick to a specific warm up and dynamic stretching prior to training and static stretching afterwards.

Each stretch should be held for approximately 10–30 seconds to the point of tightness or slight discomfort.

Repeat each stretch 2–4 times so you do around 60 seconds or longer for each stretch.

Neuro-Motor Exercise

This is a new addition to the ACSM Guidelines. Neuro-motor training is sometimes referred to by fitness professionals as functional fitness training. In fact, 'functional' is a hot word in the personal training sphere right now! Think of exercises that require balance, co-ordination, agility and gait and you're some way to understanding what we mean by functional training. I tend to explain it as lifting heavy awkward things under supervision so that when you lift heavy awkward things in real life you do it well (without injury). In many PT studios now we use ropes to pull things, we lift beer kegs full of water, run along pushing sleds, and swing kettlebells – all of this falls in the category of functional training. It is fun, challenging and exciting. It exercises the brain as well as the body.

Yoga and tai chi also fall under the category of neuro-motor exercise. It is recommended that neuro-motor exercise be done 2–3 days per week for 20–30 mins.

So, we have moved from thinking that just walking is enough in terms of exercise to a much more multi-faceted – but hopefully, more stimulating and exciting – exercise plan. A good gym or PT studio often incorporates all of these elements into the sessions they run, so shop around and find a studio which is close to home, has staff that are highly qualified, passionate and caring, and programming that is exciting. In gyms and studios, just like most things in life, you get what you pay for. There are lots of very cheap fitness centres around these days but understand that you will probably be left entirely to your own devices which can be tricky. Do a little research. Most places offer a free trial session so try before committing.

Right! You now know what you need to do and have an idea of how to get started – away you go! Let's look at a few other important aspects to help you maintain your new exercise regime for your healthy body.

Goal Setting

Keeping your eye on the prize can help enormously with motivation. Many of us work well to a timeline, so aiming for a measurable, definite goal such as a fun run can work brilliantly. Maybe your goal is to lose 5kg, or maybe it is a little more vague, 'I want to look and feel better'. Whatever your goal is, try to make it as specific and measurable as you can. For example, 'I want to look and feel better' might become:

- I want to fit back in my size 12 work clothes again
- I want to lose the belly fat – at the moment my waist is 90cm, I want to get it into the 70s
- I am so tired right now; I want to have more vim and vigour. Specifically, I'd like to have the energy to do something after dinner (e.g. go for a walk).

Self-Talk

What we say to ourselves about ourselves is extremely powerful. The sort of things people say about their training can often involve long held personal beliefs e.g.:

- I'm not a sporty person
- I'm not co-ordinated
- I'm always the last one picked for teams
- I'm an all or nothing person.

Sometimes with clients I find these statements are referring back to events from primary school! Some of the people who go on to achieve amazing fitness and physique success in my business are the very ones who earnestly told me how unsporty they were on our first meeting.

The 'all or nothing' self-talk is extremely common. It also masquerades as 'I'm either full-on or full-off', and as soon as I hear this I know some basic rethinking is needed.

In terms of exercise (and healthy eating), saying to yourself that you are all or nothing means that you are going to be full-on, going to the gym every day, eating incredibly strictly (and maybe feeling deprived) and then the slightest set back (e.g. a missed day at the gym) will mean complete derailment, and maybe throwing in the towel all together.

It can also mean that buying a packet of chocolate biscuits and eating one turns into eating six, then eating all of them and hiding the packet in the bottom of the rubbish bin and feeling guilty!

Instead of thinking of yourself as an all or nothing person, try this approach:

'I used to be an all or nothing person, now I would say I am an 80/20 person. If I have a slip up, I just let it go and resume my usual efforts. I am really forgiving of my mistakes and know to expect them from time to time. I'm in this for the long haul, so the occasional missed workout or chocolate biscuit is hardly a big deal.'

Motivation

There are two types of motivation; internal and external. People sometimes expect that motivation for exercise:

- should be there all the time
- should never vary
- is absolutely crucial to have before actually doing any exercise
- is just naturally super high in athletes, trainers and regular exercisers.

Motivation is a very fickle friend; it comes and goes. Inexplicably, you may wake up one morning and think, 'Gosh, I feel like a bike ride!' If you dig a little deeper, however, there is normally an underlying reason for this motivation. It might be:

Extrinsic:
- You have a new bike
- You have some new cycling gear
- Your cute neighbour has taken up riding
- The children really wanted to go for a ride yesterday and you couldn't.

Intrinsic:
- You feel like breathing in some fresh air and feeling alive
- It's a beautiful day and you want to get out in it
- You always feel happy after exercising.

We rarely feel motivation for no reason at all (hence the importance of goal setting)! The great thing about motivation is it is not in the lap of the gods; it is something YOU can control.

Think about the things you find motivating. It may be thinking about your friend who is in great shape and really committed to exercise and healthy eating. Connect with that friend a little more – maybe make time for a coffee once a week. Exercise people LOVE it when their friends come on board and are generally happy to help and encourage.

Perhaps it is looking at fitspo or fitspiration (yes, this is a real term) images on Pinterest and Instagram (bear in mind that these images can also be vaguely demoralising as the images are so perfect/photoshopped, etc.). There are also lots of people on social media documenting their own fitness journeys and these can be super motivating to read about.

Magazines such as *Oxygen* and *Men's Health* can also help you stay on track.

Hire a trainer (of course)! Someone who understands you, reminds you of your 'why' and guides you gently but firmly in the right direction.

Finally, and here is the clincher, DO NOT rely on motivation at all. Regard your training as you do your day job. Unless you loathe your job, most of us don't expect to be highly motivated and pumped to go to work each day – we just get up and go without a second thought. Try this approach with your training, too – book it in, go, get it done. Before you know it, it's simply a habit, a part of your day that you don't miss. Even better, before you know it, you will have made a few friends at the gym/studio who you regularly see, started noticing some physical changes, and you will feel a heap happier, less stressed and more energised. Once that habit is established and you start to see the benefits you are literally up and running!

Exercise is not an optional extra for a healthy life. It is something every one of us must get done. It is simply a question of finding a way of training that suits your lifestyle, budget and what you enjoy. Have fun with it and don't be scared of working hard – bodies love to move.

Movement is magic!

References:

Level of exercise statistics n.d., Heart Foundation, https://www.heartfoundation.org.au/about-us/what-we-do/heart-disease-in-australia/level-of-exercise-statistics

Garber, CE, Blissmer, B, Deschenes, MR, Franklin, BA, Lamonte, MJ, Lee, I, Nieman, DC 2011, 'Quantity and Quality of Exercise for Developing and Maintaining Cardiorespiratory, Musculoskeletal, and Neuromotor Fitness in Apparently Healthy Adults: Guidance for Prescribing Exercise', *Medicine & Science in Sports & Exercise*, vol.43, no.7, pp. 1334-1359

What's love got to do with it?

Mary Jo Mc Veigh

Before we delve into this chapter I invite you to pause. Pause and think of someone you love. If more than one person pops into your mind allow that to happen. See yourself doing something fun with them.

Stay with that picture for a few breaths. As you see this picture turn your attention to your body and the physical feeling of love. Focus on where you feel it in your body. If the feeling has a physical sensation stay with it. If the physical sensation is not easily accessible imagine the feeling of love as a colour, a beam of light, or gentle flowing water. Allow the sensation or the visualisation to spread and flow throughout your entire body. Slowly, gently, feel or watch it flow. Stay with this experience as long as you want before continuing to read this chapter. Notice the difference on how you felt before and after this short exercise.

Emotional Wisdom

What you have just achieved by engaging in that very simple exercise is an improvement in your physical health. It did not involve expensive medications, time-consuming exercise routines, or advice from external parties. The health benefits that you have just received emanated from within you, from the innate healing potential that lies within the powerhouse of your emotional wisdom (E.W.).

Harnessing the power of emotions for physical health is not an alternative to medical intervention, expert clinical advice, or a stable exercise routine. E.W. goes hand in hand with all other interventions available to us. Tapping into E.W. can be as big a part of your daily health practices as brushing your teeth is to good dental care or eating a balanced diet is to digestive wellbeing.

Providing training in the trauma and therapeutic field for over 20 years, I regularly facilitate preventive courses for workers to avoid burnout or vicarious trauma. One exercise I employ is to ask for a show of hands of how many people in the room clean their teeth every day. Every hand shoots up. There is no argument against the benefit of daily brushing to remove bacteria, plaque, and other nasties that compromise our dental health.

The next question is how many clean their emotional system every day. 90% quizzical looks, 3% frowns, 5% smiles, 2% hands up. These percentages are a representation of the affirmative responses commonly seen in over 20 years as a trainer. The audience is a group of professionals who work day in day out with the tragic effects of emotional dis-ease of the people who seek their assistance. These professionals know the impact of emotions on wellbeing and yet they seem to disconnect this knowing when it comes to thinking about the need for the emotional-physical fusion for health.

Emotional-Physical Fusion

Dr Candice Pert (1999) in her book, *The Molecules of Emotions*, demonstrates how emotions carry information to link the major systems of the body into one functioning unit.

When we have an external experience that evokes an emotional response the external experience becomes internalised and we name it a feeling. This 'feeling' does not enter our body as a piece of physical matter like food. Moreover, when it is in the body it does not float around as a nonentity like a little thought bubble we see in cartoon drawings. It becomes part of the physical reality of the body.

What's in Your Day?

In an average day each person is bombarded with multiple experiences, many of which have an emotional component. Whether we realise it or not we convert these emotional experiences into chemicals that flow throughout our body and effect our health (Pert 1999).

The emotional nature of each experience will activate different physical reactions in the body. Take, for example, a very simple everyday action: standing in a post office queue. If you are in a hurry and start to feel irritated at the snail pace movement of the queue, your stress system will be activated. If you have just finished lunch with someone you love and, while in the queue, replay the conversation you had during lunch and feel the same feelings of joy, you will activate the relaxation system.

Stomach

Dr Michael D. Gershon (1998), highlighted emotional aspects of bowel and intestine health. This knowledge stretches as far back as the nineteenth century to a German neurologist, Leopold Auerbach, who discovered a complex network of nerve cells, like those of the human brain, exist in the intestines.

If the stomach, intestines and bowel regions of the body were merely a biological digestion and waste disposal system the evidence of the thinking and feeling that the above experts uncovered would not exist. We would not feel 'butterflies in our tummy' when we were excited, we would not feel 'sick to our stomach' when we received bad news, we would not feel a 'knot in our stomach' when we were nervous. Unless we had the biological 'feeling' apparatus in that part of our body, we would not locate any emotional reactions to a situation there at all.

Heart

The work of the HeartMath Institute in this century modernises this message of the importance of the heart not in the word 'grace' but 'health'. Their research has highlighted that the heart is the central, rhythmic force in the body. The rhythm of the heart is known as Heart Rate Variability and displays the emotional state of a person. The HeartMath Institute propose that if the heart's rhythm is regular and reliable and stable, the rest of the body will fall into entrainment.

This reliable and stable condition is not only

achieved through good physical health but also emotional health. The more a person approaches life from a positive emotional state, the healthier their heart and hence their general health is. This is why using your E.W. is important to physical health along with others forms of knowledge such as nutrition or exercise.

Brain

From an evolutionary point of view an important aspect of human development was the ability to make vital choices between growth and connection or protection and defence. In harsh environments or in the presence of animals we needed to effectively switch between these two systems.

The limbic system is the decision maker in this survival system with a part of the brain called the amygdala being the CEO. The limbic system needs to work outside of conscious awareness to ensure survival. To put it bluntly, the part of the brain that is responsible for philosophical or existential thinking requires conscious focus and is too slow if a dangerous raging animal is hurtling towards you. This limbic system signals the body to move to defend itself in the face of danger by either freezing, fighting, or flighting from the danger.

The vehicles we jump into everyday need fuel to move us from point A to point B. Without fuel there is no movement. The body is no different and in situations of danger it particularly needs a source of energy. Cortisol is this source. It, for example, provides energy by increasing blood sugar levels, sharpens our memory to tap into recognising danger, dulls our reaction to pain and grabs calcium from our bones to give to the muscles that need to be used in freeze, fight or flight.

Short periods of cortisol activation help us to survive, but living in a state of high stress or hypervigilance to danger floods the body with cortisol. Trauma research has highlighted that high levels of cortisol affect brain development in children to the point that some clinicians speak of brain damage. In adults it has been linked to, amongst other things, type 2 diabetes, bone degeneration, hypertension and suppressed immunity.

The brain can process 400 billion bits of information a day but the average person focuses on only 2,000. Whenever we put our attention on something we are firing neurons and laying down brain circuits. So what we put our attention on is the circuit we are creating. When we are putting our attention on issues that stress us and cause us distress we are keeping the adrenal system and the cortisol production flowing. When we put our attention on issues that interest us, inspire us, and/or relax us, we are firing the neural pathways in that direction.

Relating Along the Way

Having just taken a very brief glimpse at the body from the stomach to the brain we can see that the emotional environment of the body affects physical health. Emotional and physical wellbeing are inextricably linked. So how do you create and maintain healthy emotions as part of healthy body? The answer to this lies in how you relate to all emotions that you experience and how you use your E.W. as part of your health care plan.

Relating with What is Commonly Termed the 'Negative Emotions'.

The body reacts to emotional danger in the same way it reacts to physical danger. For example, our cortisol levels rise if we have a fear of dogs regardless of whether we are near the dog or think about the dogs.

The research of the HeartMath Institute highlights that emotions that are labelled negative and situations that are stressful increase the severity of diseases and worsen the prognosis for people who have different health conditions.

The feelings associated with emotionally charged or stressful situations are detrimental to health and need to be addressed. However, they are a part of our complex survival system and should not be ignored or forced away with shallow happy thoughts. Hearing potentially life threatening news about health and then being told to think of a happy place is not only discounting a very frightening situation, it can further compound the situation by blocking natural stress reactions.

The emotions that tend to get labelled 'negative' are feelings like anger, sadness, hatred, frustration, jealousy, etc. They are more aptly named 'difficult or challenging emotions' because they *do* cause discomfort or unease within us.

'Difficult or challenging emotions' are not negative. They are part of the complexity of the human condition. They are life telling you something and wanting a response. The negative effects on you of these emotions depends on how you relate to these.

To live a healthy emotional life is to allow yourself and to be allowed by others to stay in authentic connection with the emotional experience. When someone betrays you, the feeling of revenge may rise from the pain of that experience. When you are bereft of someone you love, sadness may be the place the heart goes. When you are abused by someone, anger may course through your body. There is nothing WRONG or NEGATIVE about these feelings. They are your reactions within the context of the experience you have gone through.

Emotions as Messengers

Anger is seen as one of the feelings on top of the list of these negative emotions. If left unchecked, it can keep you in a state of hyper arousal. If acted upon in violence to another, it can cause pain and destruction. Living in a chronic state of anger or using anger to act destructively towards yourself for others is undoubtedly an emotional and physical health problem. What I propose is another way to relate to your feeling of anger when it arises. It is a way that does not act destructively or harms yourself for others. It is a way that relates to your feeling as a messenger.

What if while listening to your anger as a messenger you start to recognise a passion for a cause and see the truth of a situation that speaks to ethics of justice and human rights? What if while listening to your anger as a messenger you feel the strength to stand up for yourself and defend the dignity of your personhood?

Anger as a burning fire of passion or strength can cause great and wonderful change for the good on an individual level and a global level. The history of human rights activism was not written by complacency. The force that ignites a passion to improve the life of another is often one that lives in the fire of someone's sense of outrage at the violation of rights or abuse that people are being subjected to. It is a form of anger that is liberating, not destructive.

Sadness is another emotion that some want to shoo away or corral into neat ways of expression. Again, like anger, sadness – left without the company of your attention – can move into chronic states of despair, which cause major health problems. The hormones secreted by the adrenal gland in situations of helplessness and hopelessness depress the immune system. It inhibits the synthesis of antibodies, reducing their number and inhibiting the activity of the T cells.

However, sadness can bring us the purifier of water: tears. Tears are not only one of the body's major ways of eliminating toxins from the body, they are also a companion to our sadness. They give external physical expression to an internal lonely torment. As the salty warmth rolls down our cheek we can feel skin and water touch and so be touched by our own sadness and allow this union its time.

Until recent times the Irish had a beautiful tradition of keening at funerals. The word keening comes from the Irish verb, 'ag caoineadh' which means 'crying'. Indigenous Irish women were guardians of this ritual and they would lament in song and voice at funerals. There were no words of, 'Hush up now and stop crying.' There was, instead, a public honouring of wailing and crying and singing and giving voice to the deep sadness in grief. And when the ritual has run its course the silence that was left behind was the nest where healing could begin.

It is vital for health to give voice in whatever way that fits with your healing to the depths of all your emotions. If you approach all your difficult emotions with a sense that you should not be feeling them, then you are adding guilt to the pile.

You may then add impatience as you feel a need to change them quickly, followed with a dose of critical judgement for feeling them in the first place. Adding guilt, impatience, and criticism to a situation that already was causing some distress or discomfort silences your reality and strips away compassion for who you are. These are perfectly acceptable in your human reactions.

All feelings are evidence of a life lived. They are telling us something about the situation we find ourselves in or the experience we are going through. Listening to the 'messenger' and finding the right relationship with it is the key to emotional and physical health.

To relate to the more difficult or challenging emotions involves steps of recognition and engagement with them.

We must first acknowledge that we are feeling the emotion and then name it. This does not equate to a justification for our subsequent actions (*I feel anger therefore I am entitled to shout at you*), nor an effort to push them away (*I feel anger but should not because good people don't feel angry*). At this stage it means recognising that it is a feeling and it can be named.

When acknowledged and named we can approach it with curiosity – a curiosity that dwells in wonderment rather than forensic questioning allows us to notice how the feeling arose (because this was said or done) and the values that lie within us from this noticing (*I feel angry because I am tired and not thinking clearly* or *I feel angry because that was a great act of injustice that occurred*).

From this place of curious inquiry – that locates the feeling in a context of ethics or values or just plain momentary human fragility – we can ask if the feeling is serving us (and others). With this exploration comes movement.

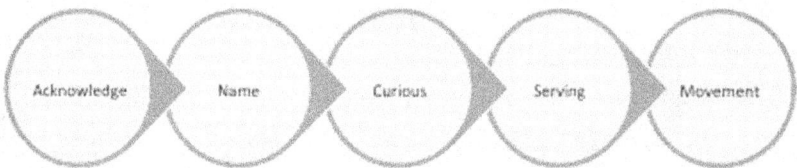

Acknowledge ▶ Name ▶ Curious ▶ Serving ▶ Movement

Movement in Thought and Body

Mc Veigh (2015, p. 45) wrote:

In the traditional Irish language, when you express a feeling you would not say that you are the feeling – for example, 'I am sad.' You would say that you are in a relationship to the feeling. For example, the sadness is upon you or you are with the sadness, or sadness is moving through you.

This linguistic and experiential reality allows the person to have a relationship with the feeling that allows for movement rather than permanency. If a feeling can come upon you then a feeling can leave.

As a result, the person experiencing the feeling can have more governance over the feeling. This is not denying the emotion, but it is engaging with it from a place of mastery rather than submission.

It is important therefore to bring movement of thought and language to the emotions that feel challenging.

Be careful not to lock yourself into the time and place of the emotion. You are not your emotions. They are the messenger in you.

Allow them the time to visit you in the experience you are going through without denying or rushing them through AND allow them to exist in the energy of movement that is recognising they will pass.

Masaru Emoto, (2001, p. xvi) said this beautifully when he wrote:

'Water in a river remains pure because it is moving. When water becomes trapped it dies. Therefore, water must constantly be circulated ... so when your emotions flow throughout your body, you feel a sense of joy and move towards physical health. Moving, changing, flowing – that is what life is all about.'

Connecting physical movement of the body with emotional movement is a great wellbeing technique. If you have ever noticed your body when a feeling like sadness or depression comes to call you may notice a hunching of the shoulders, a stoop in the back or a folding over in the torso. Feelings on the sadness end of the spectrum have a heaviness about them and the body registers this as if it is carrying a physical burden.

We talk of people who are happy as having a 'bounce in their step'. This is not just an adage; it is good advice. It is important to bring lightness and an upward movement to the body to either assist you to move the feelings on or to unburden the body when the feelings passes. Go for a walk and put a physical bounce into your step. Put on your favourite uplifting music and dance with gay abandon around your house, go swimming and feel the joy of the water move over your body and perhaps indulge in a few silly splashes while you are it.

While moving the body, be purposeful in bringing into your body the feelings you wish to feel – for example, joy or hope. You will not only invite these feelings into existence but you will boost your immune system, physically strengthen your body, and perspiration from physical exertion will help detox the body.

Using the breath is another great technique to detox the body after difficult feelings and invite the nurturing feelings into your body.

Mc Veigh (2015, p. 62) reminds us:

Much is known about the benefits of purposeful breathing. We can consciously use our breathing to affect the sympathetic and parasympathetic nervous systems. During times of emotional stress, our sympathetic nervous system is activated and affects a number of physical responses in our body.

When our body is in a state of calm homeostasis, we are more able to access the parts of the brain that control creative, philosophical or reflective thinking. A brain in hyper-arousal is designed to activate the body for survival thinking only (fight, flight or freeze). In this physical state, breathing tends to be shallower and located in the higher regions of the chest. This form of chest breathing is less efficient for optimal oxygen supply to the blood, and hence to the brain. Slower, deeper breaths use the lower lobes of the lungs and cause the greatest amount of blood flow. The most commonly known technique of breathing into the abdomen region is the one that accesses lower lung lobe breathing.

This form of breathing is well known in yogic and relaxation fields, and is a recommended practice for general health and wellbeing.

Breathing can be combined with sound, thought or image to strengthen the invitation of the feeling you wish to invoke. For example, with sound you may listen to a piece of music or create a sound on a Tibetan bowl and breathe to the rhythm of the sound.

With thought you could think about a word (peace, joy, calm, etc.) and inhale the word and exhale the emotion you are freeing yourself from (despair, revenge, etc.). With image, you could imagine a tranquil scene and breathe in the imagined peace of the scene you created.

Create and Maintain this Relationship with All Emotions that Challenge

Creating and maintaining this relationship with all emotions is vital for our health. E.W. knows how to honour the balance between challenging and the uplifting emotions is important. Mc Veigh (2016, p. 96), brings us into the wisdom of the Celts to see

'The Celtic Irish healers encouraged the seeking of balance to maintain health. This balance was seen as internal to an individual person – a balance of mind, body and spirit.'

Expression – not suppression – will create the movement needed for healing and, as time allows, the more uplifting emotions that assist us to maintain our health will visit again.

Relating with what is Commonly Termed the 'Positive Emotions'

The research of the HeartMath Institute (2015, p. 25) looked at the importance for health for what is commonly termed positive feelings:

'Positive emotions not only feel better, they actually tend to increase synchronisation of the body's systems, thereby enhancing energy and enabling us to function with greater efficiency and effectiveness.'

The positive emotions they highlighted include – amongst others – joy, appreciation, gratitude, hope, love. These mighty five in any combination or quantity are a pretty reliable recipe for good.

Joy

From her research, Sonja Lyubomirsky (2007, p. 26) concludes:

'In sum, across all the domains of life, happiness appears to have numerous positive by-products; in becoming happier we not only boost experiences of joy, contentment, love, pride and awe, but we also improve other aspects of our lives – energy levels, our immune system, our engagement with work and with other people, and our physical and mental health.'

Two neurotransmitters that are particularly associated with joy are serotonin and dopamine. Serotonin is known to boost your mood, hence it is good to have a supply on hand to increase your sense of joy. In addition, it is a great chemical ally in more difficult times. Four important activities keep your serotonin reserves stocked up through:

- developing cognitive abilities to direct your mind towards positive thinking
- exposure to sunlight
- low intensity exercise
- consumption of tryptophan with carbohydrates.

Research has highlighted the benefits of tryptophan to increase a sense of wellbeing. In particular, it is associated with assisting sleep, calming moods and dealing with anxiety. However, if you suffer from any extremes of these conditions, that is sleep deprivation, inability to self soothe or debilitating anxiety, consulting medical advice is highly recommended.

Dopamine is the neurotransmitter associated with pleasure-seeking behaviour but it is also stimulated when you feel the reward of achieving a goal. Two important considerations to release dopamine are:

- Setting achievable goals and celebrating their attainment before rushing on to the next one
- Exercising with a goal-focused orientation that is positive rather than negative. For example, change the goal from a compulsion to lose weight to a desire to feel good about yourself when you reach a certain weight.

The experience of joy is a very individual experience so this section will not conclude with a list of activities to make you feel happy. Having a relationship with what makes *you* feel joy is the important key to unlocking the necessary neurotransmitters.

It may not necessarily be about doing lots of activities or owning lots of things. Indeed, it may be the opposite. But it is important to give some thoughtful consideration to it as part of your physical health plan.

One of the exercises I do on the preventive emotional health training courses I conduct for professionals is a sensory audit. Recently, a young woman spoke about loving the smell of coriander as it reminded her of her grandmother.

As she spoke, the young woman was animated and smiling and when asked how she felt having the conversation she said she felt great joy. She was not sitting beside her grandmother, yet she was present to the joy (and love) she felt for her. In that moment, the young woman was not only emotionally feeling joy, she was – according to research – improving her physical health (for example, boosting her immune system).

When I asked if she grew coriander she said no as firstly she had no garden and secondly did not like the taste of it in food. I inquired what it would be like if she kept a pot of it on her kitchen window and, on days when she was having a tough time, crushed them to release the aroma.

After a momentary pause and a gentle stream

of tears, she said she would love that as she would be back in her grandmother's arms and she would feel happy again. At the end of the training, the young woman spoke to me about the struggles she was currently going through and how this simple act could help her. She spoke as if she had been given the code to unlock some eternal secret. It is not a mystical act that I performed as a trainer. It was a simple act of demonstrating conscious movement towards joy, using an aspect of E.W. that is accessible to all of us.

Keeping joy in your life is not a flippant pursuit of happiness. It requires purposeful awareness about your life and your part in living a life that contains joy. It is engaging in meaningful acts and being with people (in body or thought) who are dear to you.

Moreover, for your physical health it involves knowing your source of joy at its deepest level and bringing it close to you so you can call upon it at the most difficult times.

Invitation to Pause

Pause to notice what brings joy into your life. If joy is ever-present take time to celebrate this further in your thoughts. If joy is in short supply make a commitment to yourself to do one thing in the next week that will make you feel joyous.

Appreciation

Appreciation of natural beauty is a vital form of building health. Being exposed to images of beauty and engaging in practices of beauty build neural pathways that lead to a more positive view of the world. The more positive and hopeful the view of the world, the more you release the neurotransmitters associated with happiness.

Berman, Jonides, and Kapla (2008) found an increase in performance on memory and attention after research participants went for a walk in an arboretum. In addition, they found that showing images of nature, while not producing the same level of improved functions, did show an increase in memory performance and attention.

Studies (Ulrich, R.S., 1984; Ulrich, R.S. & Lunden, O. 1990) discovered that patients with views of nature had quicker and easier recovery times from surgery.

Being in nature as well as appreciating it has multiple health benefits, especially if you are barefoot. Ober, Sinatra, and Zucker (2014) explored how reconnecting the body to the earth (earthing) has multiple health benefits. In their book they comprehensively explored how:

'Earthing is among the most natural and safest things you can do to improve your health; something simple yet astoundingly profound. It is not a treatment but a hugely rewarding return-to-a-core aspect of Nature that we have abandoned. Earthing is a missing link in the earth equation.'
(Ober, C., Sinatra, S.T., & Zucker, M. 2014, p. 5)

The way to this health improvement can be as simple as walking or sitting on the land every day barefoot.

Invitation to Pause

Pause to notice what images of beauty you have in your life, how often you are in the natural environment, and what you do to bring beauty into your life. If beauty is ever-present or you walk barefoot or spend time in nature, take time to celebrate this further in your thoughts. If beauty is in short supply or you have never walked barefoot or spend little time in nature, make a commitment to yourself to do one thing in the next week that will change this and build up from there.

Hope

In the therapeutic world that I work in, research has shown that procedures, techniques and therapeutic rituals that inspire hope in clients and have a positive expectation for change will lead to change.

The use of hope for healing does not live in the realm of therapy alone. It is an emotional technology available to us all as a very powerful resource for health. In terms of physical health, it has been shown that living in a chronic state of hopelessness or helplessness compromises the immune system. The hormone secreted by the adrenal gland in these situations inhibits the synthesis of antibodies, reducing the number and inhibiting the activity of the T cells. The T cells are the body's soldiers in the fight against disease.

The most important aspect of using hope as a resource for good physical health is to realise that hope is not just an emotion.

Hope can also be a choice that turns into action.

As a choice, hope means that you do not bury your head in the sand or cling to false beliefs. It means choosing to face each challenge that throws itself in front of you with a hope-filled attitude that will benefit you, and *not* lead you into despair. From this place of hope, action can be taken to realise a better way forward.

It is a choice that one person took when faced with double amputation of his legs. He did not say he hoped for his legs to grow back – this is a biological impossibility. He said, 'I hope to walk again', and he did on prosthetic legs. His choice led to his actions that required hours of fittings and readjustments, specialised psychotherapy and daily exercise.

Hope that is anchored in everyday life leads to authentic choices that can keep you motivated to live in a fuller and healthier way. It requires routines and rituals that keep you in the habit of choosing hope over despair. Once good habits are established, it is harder to break them when life circumstances invite you away from them.

Invitation to Pause

Pause to notice your relationship with
hope. If hope is ever-present take time to
celebrate this further in your thoughts.
If hope is in short supply make a
commitment to yourself to do one thing
in the next week that will bring hope into
your life.

Gratitude

It is important to know what definition of gratitude
we are working with before seeking to unlock the
benefits of it. The definition of gratitude referred to
is not found in fleeting moments of thankfulness.
While momentary thankfulness is important as
a form of social cohesion, relationship-building
and a sign of social skills, it is not this form of
gratitude that bolsters health.

Gratitude that affirms beneficence in life despite
the circumstances of life and acknowledges a
source to be thankful to is the form of gratitude
that is linked to health benefits. Being in this state
of gratitude means that the person approaches
life with acceptance, an abundance attitude, and
grateful thinking as their cognitive default button.

The power of gratitude for increased health
benefits has attracted increasing scientific
attention. Research in this area has shown
gratitude to have emotional and physical health
benefits.

The physical benefits for health are, for example:

- decrease in suffering from common aches and pains in the body
- lower blood pressure
- increased energy to exercise
- strengthened immune system
- deeper and longer sleep, and awaking rested
- giving more attention to a better health care plan.

Research on the characteristics of people who are grateful shows they are happier, hopeful, forgiving, do good deeds and are connected to others.

Invitation to Pause

Pause to notice your relationship with gratitude and the above characteristics. If you are strong in these areas take time to celebrate this further in your thoughts. If not, make a commitment to yourself to do one thing in the next week that will strengthen you living life in a state of gratitude.

LOVE

The most common thinking about love is of love as a feeling. The feeling of love can mean to have a tenderness or friendship towards someone; it can mean having a liking or preference for an object or activity, or it can mean having an erotic attraction to a lover. These are all very different feelings and are as dependent on who or what is receiving the love as it does on the engendering of this feeling.

Love, as a feeling, has a physical sensation in the body and can be evoked not just in the presence of the person or object of your love but in the thought of them. The invocation of the thought that leads to the feeling of love is a very powerful gateway to activating the production of the neurotransmitters discussed earlier that are associated with joy and hence unlocking the health benefits related to them.

Love is also a call to action. It invites the consideration of how to act lovingly on behalf of oneself or to another, and how to do the work of love for the betterment of self or other. This calls for a depth of E.W. that notices thoughts and actions that are deprecating or destructive of self or others. It invites placing our attention on these thoughts and actions and redirecting them to more life-affirming and nurturing ways.

Invitation to Pause

Pause to notice any habitual thoughts or
actions that are deprecating or destructive
of self or others and ask yourself these
questions:

- What would love say to me?
- What would love want me to do?

References

Berman, MG, Jonides, J, Kapla, S 2008, 'The
cognitive benefits of interacting with nature',
*Psychological Science: A journal of the American
Psychology Society,* vol.19, no.12, pp. 1207-1212.

Emotos, M 2008, *The Hidden Messages in Water,*
Beyond Words Publishers, Oregon.

Gershon, MD 1998, *The second brain: A ground-
breaking new understanding of nervous disorder of
the stomach and intestine,* Harper Collins, New
York.

Lyubomirsky, S 2008, *The How of Happiness. A
scientific approach to getting the life you want,* The
Penguin Press, New York.

Mc Veigh, MJ 2013, *Discovering Audacious Love,*
Balboa Press, Bloomington.

Mc Veigh, MJ 2015, *Without Question. The language
of Leadership,* Busybird Publishing, Victoria.

Mc Veigh, MJ 2015, 'Sacred Harmony', *Healthy Mind*, Busybird Publishing, Victoria, pp. 81-101.

Ober, C, Sinatra, ST, Zucker, M 2014, *Earthing. The most important discovery ever*, Basic Health Publications, CA.

Pert, C 1999, *The Molecules of Emotion. The science behind mind body medicine*, Touchstone Publisher, New York.

Keniger, LE, Gaston, KJ, Irvine, KN, Fuller, RA 2013, 'What are the benefits of

interacting with nature?', *International Journal of Environmental Research & Public Health*, vol.10, no.3, pp. 913-35.

Townsend, M 2013, 'Health Benefits of Nature', *International Journal of Environmental Research & Public Health.*

Ulrich, RS 1984, 'View from a window may influence recovery form surgery' *Science*, vol.224, pp. 420-421.

Ulrich, RS, Lunden, O 1990, 'Effects of nature and abstract pictures on patients recovering form open heart surgery', paper presented at the International Congress of Behavioural Medicine, Uppslaa, Sweden, June 27-30.

pharmacist

The Alchemy of
Optimal Health

Vanita Dahia

If you had unlimited resources in time, money and food, what would great health look like to you? Every day, patients trickle into doctor's and health provider's rooms to look for a Band-Aid quick fix. They wait and wait for that prescription. The waiting room is often lined with old magazines.

If airports can become shopping malls and McDonald's playgrounds, should clinics have health-associated distractions like a treadmill or food preparation demonstrations?

We have the presumption that a headache may be cured with a pill. Instead, we owe it to ourselves to investigate upstream and enquire upon the clinical drivers. Are the headaches relieved with drinking more water, removing sugars or caffeine? Or could it be associated with the mould or water leaks in the house?

What does good health look like?

To illustrate this, I'll tell you about Jane. She went to her doctor with premenstrual syndrome (PMS), low libido, weight gain and mood swings. She was concerned about her lack of libido as she was dabbling in the dating scene. She had been prescribed an antidepressant for her PMS.

Teri Pearlstein and Meir Steiner have reported in the Journal of Psychiatry and Neuroscience, 2008 that selective serotonin reuptake inhibitors

(SSRI's) are effective for premenstrual dysphoric disorder (PMDD). Jane felt better initially on the SSRI, but gained weight with prolonged use. She could not shift the weight and reported feeling like a 'zombie' described as being emotionally flat.

Despite Dr Google's assistance, she needed help in digging deeper into her chemistries to find the underlying cause of hormonal dysregulation, if that was in fact to blame.

She discovered that the innate, fundamental body's expression of optimal health is vitality and well-being. This is a state of a sound, highly-functioning body and a joyful state of the mind.

Optimal health is defined by the Constitution of the World Health Organisation as a state of complete physical, mental and social well-being and not merely the absence of disease or infirmity.

The alchemy of optimal health is an amazing body, remarkable physiology, a limitless mind, and an eternal spirit that is sensitive to thoughts, feelings and the environment. At any given moment, the cells in the body adjust by releasing chemicals that affect the physiology, emotions and the genes.

Natural healing capacity of the body occurs with full engagement of the powerful mechanisms of biochemistry and energetic transformation to promote self-healing at a molecular level.

The basis of disease is disruption of the internal regenerative and healing mechanisms. The wide variety of healing approaches from nutrition, herbs, pharmaceuticals, mind-body medicine, to fitness and health promotion have something in common: they identify the underlying causes of disharmony or disease and the opportunity for the body to bring things back into alignment.

Transformation of the medical model can only shift to the mental model. Life is experience which can only be regulated by what we think or feel. In the context of healing, health is not a pill. Medical parameters are necessary but should not be overridden by opening the inner dimension of the mind.

Health could be expressed as pleasantness of the body and joy as the pleasantness of the mind. Extreme pleasantness of the mind may be expressed as an emotion such as love, compassion or bliss. When your surroundings and environment are pleasant, we may have success, whereas inner pleasantness is 100% ours.

The body is programmed for health. Illness can be categorised into two types: infectious or chronic. External invasion of microbes leading to infections can most effectively be treated through the conventional or naturopathic antimicrobial systems. More than 70% of ailments are self-created within you. These are chronic ailments such as heart conditions, depression, diabetes, obesity, cancer and so on.

If we are creating chronic conditions within us, we need to therefore fix or quell the illness from within. Why would the cells in the body turn against you? We start incubating misunderstandings at a cellular level, hence need to activate the inner energy and get access to a deeper dimension of intelligence from within.

There is no need to chemically bomb the body when sick, instead we need to listen and act on the emotional attachment associated with physical illness or outcome.

In essence, illness is a physiological manifestation of imbalance from within, for which the mind is the master controller. From a biochemical basis, the chemistry of physiology is controlled by the chemistry of the mind.

The most sophisticated piece of equipment on the planet is our body and mind. The body turns food into human cells. If there is an illness, don't go to the local tinker, go to the manufacturer!

For long-term health, dial up the concept of health from the inside, which can change the chemistry of the mind and body within weeks. Most of the work is done when optimising diet, lifestyle and exercise by balancing gut, adrenal and hormone function.

Jane started a regular exercise routine. She also joined a belly dancing class as the regular warming effect of pelvic movement assisted in period pain.

The brain systems involved in the matter of sex drive is governed by the most primitive part of the limbic system which drives emotions, relationships and romance.

Sex drive is often associated with testosterone. Well, the body is not so simplistic. Sexual traits and libido can be best classified into four brain system drivers.

Modern dating sites use these systems to

match participants based on their personalities and traits. The drivers of libido or partner choice may be expressed as:

- Dopamine driver, which is a reward and satisfaction neurotransmitter. The typical characteristics are creativity, expressivity, curiosity and spontaneity. These are people who are drawn to others a bit like themselves.

- The next driver is serotonin, the happy brain chemical. These are people who tend to be traditional, follow the rules, like order, authority and may be religious. They seek people with similar interests.

- The other two drivers are oestrogen and testosterone, sex hormones that represent logical directness, decisiveness, communication, and are emotionally expressive, need nurturing, and may be intuitive. These are people who tend to seek the opposite traits in their partner.

The paradox of choice when travelling upstream to hormones and neurotransmitters!

How does low sex drive, dating, moods and PMS affect Jane's chemistry?

The endocrine system controls sex hormones, the ability to cope with stress, regulates temperature, and controls metabolism. Any imbalances in the system lead to many chronic conditions. Hormones like cortisol, oestrogen, progesterone, leptin, insulin, serotonin, testosterone and others are affected by diet, lifestyle, exercise, sleep habits and weight. When these hormones are out of whack, you might need to replenish the missing hormones in conjunction with adjusting your diet, mind and lifestyle. Hormones operate like an orchestra in tune: when one hormone goes out of balance, it has the potential to throw the whole orchestra out of tune. A healthy libido does not start with organs down under, it starts with desire in the brain. All these hormones talk to brain chemicals to incite desire, love and lust.

A healthy balance of hormones like oxytocin, testosterone and progesterone are needed for a great sex life and, to a lesser extent, oestrogens, dopamine and vasopressin. Oestrogens can increase serotonin, the happy hormone levels. Stress drives the stress hormone, cortisol, up which will stimulate the need for sugar and salt cravings and block serotonin. Stress therefore leads to weight gain and sad moods.

PMS may be associated with an imbalance of female hormones, oestrogen and progesterone. These fluctuate throughout the month or cyclically. When progesterone plummets relative to oestrogens, the body may become oestrogen dominant. The dip in progesterone then drives down GABA, a relaxing and calming neurotransmitter. Oestrogen dominance enhances the fluid retention, weight gain and can make Jane feel pretty irritable or irrational.

You might do all the right things – eat healthily, exercise regularly – yet the body is unhealthy!

The first step is to examine the clusters of

symptoms to establish the clinical trigger. Investigate the laboratory findings that validate the variants as you walk through the clinical door. This can be achieved with various checklists or laboratory tests which will validate the body's physiological imbalance.

If you're moody and bloated before your menstrual cycle, examine hormonal and neurotransmitter levels.

Put the pieces of the puzzle together. Understand the underlying etiology. Diagnostic criteria need to go beyond the five minute doctor appointments, Band-Aid symptom therapy, or the diagnostic statistical manual (DSM) model for mental health. We need to establish the underlying causes and clinical triggers of ill-health.

A low level of progesterone typically seen in PMS can:

- deplete the calming and relaxing neurotransmitter, GABA, manifesting in agitation, moods and anxiety
- lower serotonin, your happy hormone, manifesting as low mood
- lower dopamine and dominate oestrogens manifesting as breast tenderness
- lower beta-endorphins manifesting as cravings for sweet foods, cramps and period pain

It is clear that hormones talk to the brain chemicals.

We therefore need to choose the holistic or integrative approach, not compartmentalise the body with the psychiatrist, gastroenterologist or endocrinologist. As one untangles ill-health, one needs to bring all the tools to manage the mind, address the clusters of symptoms of other organ systems, and switch on genes like light switches with nutrigenomics, the nutrient expression of genes whilst keeping the diet, lifestyle and exercise in check.

Jane put the basic fundamentals of good diet, exercise and lifestyle into action.

Diet plays a major role in production of brain chemicals. The fundamental building blocks of nutritional metabolism is our relationship with food. It's the sum total of our innermost thoughts and feelings, it's about what we eat. The brain uses more than 60% of nutrients from the diet to cope with stress and mental health. More food is needed when stressed or depressed.

The body knows when it's out of balance. You might have sleep issues, gain weight, lose hair, become moody, lose focus or feel flat. A good, balanced diet is one of the key influences as you are what you eat. A diet rich in a variety of wholefood, plant-based options, fruits and vegetables, protein and lots of water is recommended.

After all, good mood brain chemicals are made from essential amino acids and vitamins found in protein and green leafy vegetables.

It's best to choose foods that reach gut hormones to allow you to feel fuller for longer. These are foods that are high in protein, such as fish and chicken, and low in glycaemic index (GI) like pasta, lentils and basmati rice.

Increase dopamine, the feel good hormone, with foods rich in amino acids tyrosine and phenylalanine which manufacture dopamine. These foods include fish, eggs, spirulina, beetroot, apples, kale, oregano, bananas, strawberries and green tea. Herbs such as ginkgo biloba, nettles, dandelion, and ginseng also contain tyrosine and phenylalanine. Gingko can increase dopamine while enhancing oxygen flow and blood flow to the brain.

The basis for an ideal diet is eating sufficiently with the right blend of components. When it comes to diet choices, it's overwhelming and conflicting due to the many diet options available. It is essential to get the right type and amount of foods to support a healthy lifestyle.

An ideal diet focuses on providing all the nutrients that your body needs. It comprises of macronutrients like protein, carbohydrates and fat along with micronutrients, which include vitamins and minerals. Each of them have different roles to play in maintaining various body functions.

Keep a healthy mind, exude joy and happiness by managing the mind with focused consciousness.

The inner dimension is an unchartered terrain. Your joy, agony, love and misery lies in your perception, in alignment of the mind and the body. Optimal health starts with a healthy mind. We humans are so smart; we fly to the moon and back but have difficulty in managing the mind. Mindfulness and regular meditation are effective strategies to manage the mind.

Psychotherapy, meditation and mind-body medicine plays a vital role in mental health today. In recent years, there has been a burgeoning interest in integration of Western psychotherapy techniques and Eastern meditative traditions.

Versions of meditation have had their roots in ancient Buddhism and Indian medicine for thousands of years, traditionally focusing on attainment of enlightenment. Skeptics will advocate a specific form of psychotherapy against another and meditators will do the same.

After all, your energy flows where your attention goes!

Regular exercise helps mood in so many ways. These may include:

- release of feel-good brain chemicals such as neurotransmitters, endorphins and endocannabinoids
- reduction of immune system chemicals
- improvement of circulation
- detoxification of the body
- increase of body temperature

Find the metabolic blocks by assessing and correcting the chemistries. The value of therapy must go beyond the conventional pharmaceutical model. Albeit essential for chronic complex conditions and acute infections, pharmaceutical drugs have their limitations.

They may be expensive, or require a doctor's

prescription, and they do come with their own range of side effects, adverse reactions and contra-indications especially when mixed with other drugs. Some may be prescribed one drug to counter the side effects of another, leading to a poly-pharmacy cocktail of drugs.

Complementary medicine in the guise of herbs, vitamins, minerals and amino acids together with a range of physical therapies is a growing and burgeoning market today as the consumer is becoming aware of the therapeutic value of targeted natural therapy.

Albeit much safer than drugs, natural medicine has its own set of drawbacks. They may take longer to be effective, may interact with drugs or may need more than one supplement to address the condition.

The traditional use of the age-old system of natural medicines has been used since man existed with its own flavor based on cultural traditions.

Modern medicine is embracing the science-based validity of natural medicine under the banner of integrative, compounded, holistic or functional medicine and finally valuing the efficacy and efficiency of the humble herb.

A herb such as vitex agnus cactus, also known as chasetree, has been shown in a study by Atmaca and team[1] that it improved mood

1. Teri Pearlstein and Meir Steiner, J Psychiatry Neurosci. 2008 Jul; 33(4): 291–301, Premenstrual dysphoric disorder Atmaca1 et al, Hum Psychopharmacol Clin Exp 2003; 18: 191–195, Fluoxetine versus Vitex agnus castus

comparable to a popular SSRI, Fluoxetine. Vitex is a major progesterogenic herb useful in PMS as it is capable of:

- alleviating anxiety by stimulating GABA
- supporting low mood with serotonin
- assisting in breast tenderness via dopamine support
- reducing pain sensitivity and cravings via beta-endorphin production

Vitamins are equally important. B group vitamins, especially vitamin B6, are essential for hormone and neurotransmitter production. They have been shown to improve energy, oxygenation, regulate periods and assist with moods.

Amino acids play a vital role as precursors to neurotransmitter production. We need tryptophan rich foods such as eggs, cheese, tofu, salmon, turkey, seeds and nuts to manufacture, together with vitamin B6, the happy hormone, serotonin.

You don't have to live with symptoms. The real fact is that suffering is unnecessary – it is not caused by bad luck. You may want to blame your genes. Yes, you'll need to live with your genes as they are what your parents have passed on to you. You can, however, change your genetic expression strategically with nutrigenomics.

Jane changed her diet, took some supplements and herbs, started exercising, and within one cycle was able to alleviate many symptoms. For her, the results were dramatic! She started to lose the fluid retention and weight, and dramatically increased her energy. Her mood stabilised and her libido started creeping back on track.

Consider the systems approach of integrative and functional medicine. Treat the body as a whole, address the causes and help the body to repair and heal to regain its innate physiological balance. Once this is done and dusted, the body's natural intelligence will take care of the rest.

Better Teeth, Better Health

Jonathan Chang

You've all been to a dental clinic before, so you know the drill. After being greeted by the dental assistant, you're guided into a cold white-walled room and seated in the dreaded dental chair. You're given dark glasses and a bib, the seat is laid back flat, and in walks the dentist. They introduce themselves, dribble out some small talk then ask you to open your mouth wide to be examined. Silence. As each passing moment goes by, you wonder 'Did I brush my teeth properly this morning?' or 'I hope he can't smell last night's garlic bread'. All going well, the dentist will clean your teeth and tell you to keep up the good work for the next six months until you see each other and repeat.

Through accurate promotion and education, patients can be made aware of the significant impact oral health can have on general health, well-being, and quality of life. Risk factors for bad oral health include poor diet and hygiene, trauma, stress, smoking and alcohol use. These are also common risk factors for other chronic diseases.

Good oral health can be characterised by adequate dentition and the absence of untreated tooth decay or periodontal disease and a number of other less prevalent oral diseases and disorders. A healthy mouth enables people to eat, speak and socialise without pain, discomfort or embarrassment.

The two major diseases, which affect oral health are:

1. *Dental caries (tooth decay)* wherein the breakdown of tooth structure by the activities of bacteria result in cavities or holes in teeth

2. *Periodontal (gum)* disease wherein inflammation of the gums result in destruction of the tissues and bone surrounding and supporting the teeth.

Like many areas of the body, your mouth is teeming with bacteria, the majority of which are harmless. Oral bacteria use the breakdown of sugar (mainly sucrose) in foods to make acids. These acids can attack the tooth, creating decay leading to cavitation. Hard-to-reach areas are the most commonly affected areas, such as the grooves (fissures) of teeth and in between the teeth. Primary treatment of the tooth cavity involves removal of the decay and placement of a filling (restoration). More advanced decay may necessitate a crown, root canal treatment or, if the damage is beyond repair, tooth removal (extraction).

Oral bacteria constantly form a sticky, colourless film known as *plaque* on teeth. Normally the body's natural defences and good oral health care, such as daily brushing and flossing, can remove the plaque and keep these bacteria under control. Plaque that is not removed hardens and forms *calculus,* which normal brushing can't remove and requires professional cleaning by a dental professional.

The longer plaque and calculus remain on teeth, the more harmful they become. The mildest form of gum disease is *gingivitis,* which is characterised by red, swollen and bleeding gums. It can usually be reversed with daily brushing and flossing. This form of gum disease does not result in any loss of bone and tissue supporting teeth.

If gingivitis is left untreated, it can progress to *periodontitis,* meaning inflammation around the tooth. In this advanced form, gums pull away from the tooth, forming spaces (called *pockets*) that fill with bacteria and become infected. The body's immune system fights the bacteria as the infection advances and grows below the gum line. Bacterial toxins and the body's natural response to the infection causes breakdown of the bone and tissue that support the teeth. If left untreated, the bones, gums and tissue that hold the teeth in place are destroyed. Teeth that are otherwise healthy and functional may become loose and require removal.

Periodontal disease is one of the most common diseases, which, if left untreated, becomes serious and destructive chronic infection. Smoking and diabetes are well established risk factors for periodontal disease. Stress has also been linked, but it is not clear whether the relationship has a physiological basis or is due simply to the fact that individuals under stress are less likely to maintain adequate oral hygiene.

The majority of tooth decay and gum diseases can be prevented through proper oral hygiene practices as well as avoidance of behavioural and environmental risk factors on the part of the individual.

There are several other important oral conditions, which can have an impact on general health and well-being:

- Oral cancer
- Halitosis (bad breath)
- Tooth wear
- Mouth ulcers
- Cold sores
- Dental trauma (damage of teeth due to injury)
- Tooth sensitivity

Oral Cancer

Oral cancer can affect any part of the mouth, but is most commonly found on the tongue, floor of the mouth, lips and cheeks. It has been reported that it is the sixth most common cancer in males worldwide. Symptoms of oral cancer include, but are not limited to:

- A non-healing ulcer or sore
- Red or white patches within the mouth
- A lump in the mouth or neck
- Thickening or hardening of the cheek or tongue

- Difficulty chewing, swallowing or moving the tongue
- A persistently sore throat and hoarseness
- Persistent nosebleeds and nasal congestion
- Unexplained loose teeth

Common risk factors include:

- Tobacco use – the risk of developing cancer increases with the length of time a person has smoked and the amount they have smoked
- Exposure to human papilloma virus (HPV), which has been linked to cancer of the throat and tonsils
- Consuming alcohol
- Overexposure to sunlight, increasing the risk of cancer of the lip

The key to preventing oral cancer is to not use tobacco, and to adopt a sensible approach to the consumption of alcohol. It is estimated that at least 75% of oral cancers could be prevented by eliminating tobacco use and reducing alcohol consumption.

Consider using a lip balm containing sun protection while outdoors and always maintain a healthy diet. Overall, it is vital to attend regular dental check-ups, regardless of whether you have no teeth or wear dentures.

Halitosis

Bad breath, known as *halitosis*, is considered socially unacceptable. Self-diagnosis, however, is difficult as it is not possible to easily detect an odour from one's own breath, and as such, it is not until someone tells them of odour, that they realise they have halitosis. This can cause the person stress, wondering if they smell.

Halitosis is caused primarily by excessive amounts of volatile sulphur compounds (VSCs) being produced by oral bacteria. The level of VSCs in a person's breath can vary greatly during the day and influenced by activities such as eating, drinking, oral hygiene, sleeping and effect these factors have on saliva flow.

Many individuals suffer from unpleasant breath in the morning prior to breakfast and tooth brushing. This can be attributed to the fact that saliva incubates bacteria in the mouth during sleep when saliva flow is reduced.

Systemic diseases such as diabetes, liver cirrhosis and kidney failure can also give rise to particular bad odours in the breath. While tobacco and certain foods (e.g. garlic, onion, coffee) also influence breath, their effects come from the lungs rather than the mouth itself.

Halitosis can be reduced in several ways. Oral hygiene products aimed at controlling dental caries and periodontal disease will also help prevent halitosis. Tooth brushing, tongue cleaning and chewing gum are also effective in the control of halitosis to an acceptable level.

Tooth Wear

The term *tooth wear* is used to describe the progressive loss of tooth structure due to actions other than those causing tooth decay or dental trauma. Tooth wear increases with age, and has been shown to be more prevalent in males. As people are now retaining their natural teeth into old age, the amount of tooth wear currently seen is significantly higher than in the past. Tooth wear is classified as abrasion, attrition or erosion.

Abrasion is the progressive loss of tooth structure caused by physical activity other than chewing or tooth-to-tooth contact. The primary cause is an incorrect brushing technique, resulting in grooves where the crown meets the root of the tooth. Long-term presence of tongue jewellery has also been known to cause tooth abrasion.

Attrition is the gradual loss of tooth structure caused by chewing or grinding between opposing teeth. The extent of attrition depends on the use to which an individual puts their teeth. For example, people who clench or grind their teeth (a condition known as bruxism) will experience increased attrition. Bruxism is generally a subconscious activity, occurring mainly during sleep.

Erosion is the progressive loss of tooth structure by chemical or acid dissolution in the absence of bacteria. Tooth erosion is mostly the result of frequent and excessive consumption of carbonated drinks and fruit juices with high acid levels, and is most prevalent in teenagers and young adults. Erosion is also evident in patients suffering from gastro-oesophageal reflux disease (GORD) and from certain eating disorders (e.g. anorexia, bulimia).

Adopting a correct brushing technique can greatly reduce abrasion. Importantly, vigorous horizontal scrubbing actions with a medium-hard toothbrush should be avoided, and teeth should not be used as a tool to grip or hold items. Toothpastes vary in their level of abrasiveness; whilst abrasive toothpastes help remove staining, they may also contribute to tooth wear. Individuals with signs of abrasion are advised to seek a less abrasive toothpaste.

Attrition is a slow-progressing condition and the majority of people are only made aware of this condition upon visiting the dentist. In the case of bruxism, the dentist may recommend a night guard (or splint) during sleep. In severe cases where patients experience headaches and/or difficulty opening their mouth (known as trismus), a referral to a dental specialist or physiotherapist may be required.

Reducing the frequency and intake of carbonated drinks and fruit juices can prevent tooth erosion. Tooth brushing immediately after consuming acidic drinks or food should be avoided for a period of at least 20 minutes, as the acid weakens the enamel making it susceptible to damage from brushing.

Cold Sores

Herpes simplex virus (HSV) is the responsible for cold sores. The primary oral infection typically occurs at a young age without symptoms. The skin surrounding the mouth may be affected, along with swollen lymph glands, fever and loss of appetite. After the primary oral infection,

HSV may remain dormant, only to be activated later in life as the more common herpes labialis, or *cold sores*. This reactivation can be triggered by sunlight, trauma, stress, tiredness and menstruation. An episode of cold sores usually begins with a burning sensation on the affected area of the lips, followed by painful blisters. The appearance of cold sores is a localised cluster of small vesicles along the red border of the lip or adjacent skin. These vesicles rupture, ulcerate and crust within a couple of days and resolve within 10 days. Cold sores are contagious and strict hygiene should be adopted when a person is infected.

Prevention of cold sores is difficult. A well-established ointment (containing 5% acyclovir), if applied early during the burning phase, has been effective in reducing the duration of the episode.

Mouth Ulcers

Millions of people worldwide suffer from recurrent mouth ulcers, which are often very painful. The most common presentation is *minor aphthous ulceration* (MIAU) and is most prevalent in teenagers. MIAU usually presents as one to five small ulcers (less than 1mm in diameter) on the inside of lips or cheeks, tongue or floor of mouth, and mainly located towards the front of the mouth. These ulcers are painful, especially if they involve the tongue, interfering with eating and speech. Prior to the ulceration, patients may experience a burning or prickling sensation. The ulcers may last between a few days to two weeks, most resolving within 10 days. Mild trauma from sports injuries or a rough filling can also cause ulcers. *Major aphthous ulceration* (MJAU), a more serious form of oral ulceration, affects any part of the oral cavity, including the soft palate and tonsils. The ulcers seen in MJAU are larger and can last up to a few months.

Mouth ulcers can also be the result of stress, illness, hormonal changes, menstruation and deficiencies in vitamin B12 (pernicious anaemia), iron and folic acid. Other causes of mouth ulceration include herpes infection, irritable bowel syndrome (IBS) and various immune disorders.

Adequate oral hygiene maintenance will reduce the likelihood of secondary infection when ulcers are present, though this can be difficult as patients may find tooth brushing too painful. Overnight topical steroid coverings (containing triamcinolone acetonide) can provide relief, though they can be difficult to apply and keep in place, particularly on the tongue due to constant movement and saliva flow. Local anaesthetic lozenges and ointments have been used to provide temporary pain relief when eating.

Dental Trauma

The upper central incisors are the most common teeth damaged due to an accident. Damage can range from a small enamel chip to a complicated fracture involving the nerve of the tooth (the pulp). Occasionally, the tooth can also be displaced (subluxated) or in rare instance, completely knocked out (avulsed). Dental trauma can result in long-term aesthetic, financial and functional problems for patients.

The majority of dental trauma is the result of accidents during normal everyday activities and as such prevention in these circumstances is difficult. It is recommended for people to wear mouthguards or helmets with face shields during contact sports to reduce the likelihood of injuries to the head, teeth and neck. The wearing of safety helmets (e.g. for cycling, skiing) and of car seat belts is also recommended. When tooth trauma does occur, it is important to seek immediate advice from a dental professional.

What To Do if a Tooth Gets Knocked Out?

In the instance that a deciduous (baby) tooth is knocked out completely, parents should make no attempt to replant the tooth, as this could cause the tooth to fuse to the socket, resulting in future difficulties when it comes time for the tooth to be shed. Furthermore, it can damage the permanent (adult) tooth developing under the gum. Dental advice should be sought immediately.

In the case of a permanent tooth being knocked out completely:

1. Check that the tooth is a permanent tooth – baby teeth should not be replanted.
2. Keep the injured person calm.
3. Pick up the tooth by the crown (the chewing surface) – **NOT the root.**
4. If the tooth is dirty, gently rinse the tooth in milk or saline solution such as contact lens solution for a few seconds only – **do NOT use water or scrub.**

5. If the person is conscious, hold the cleaned tooth by the crown and replace it into its socket using light pressure. In many cases, it will slip right in. Make sure it's facing the right way – **do NOT force it into the socket.**

6. Once repositioned, hold the tooth in place by getting the person to gently bite on a handkerchief or piece of gauze.

7. If the tooth cannot be replanted immediately, it can be carried inside the injured person's mouth between the teeth and inside of the cheek or in milk - do not let the tooth become dry – **do NOT use water.**

8. Seek immediate dental treatment, consider phoning ahead to tell them you are on your way.

Tooth Sensitivity

Some people suffer sudden sharp bursts of pain when consuming cold food or drinks; a condition is known as *cervical dentine sensitivity*. This is caused by exposure of the root surface of the tooth at the gum margin, which can be reactive to temperature. Cervical dentine sensitivity can be the result of gum disease, gum recession or an aggressive brushing technique with a hard toothbrush.

Similar precautions taken to prevent gum disease and tooth abrasion will also help reduce the incidence of cervical dentine sensitivity, though often it is necessary to seek advice from a dentist. The dentist may apply a topical desensitising agent to the site to alleviate the discomfort, and recommend an additional over-the-counter topical cream for daily home use. It is worth noting that tooth sensitivity can also be the result of other factors such as a cracked or leaking filling, hence the importance of seeking dental advice. In response to the ever-increasing amount of tooth wear and sensitivity, several toothpastes formulated to reduce sensitivity are now on the commercial market.

How Does Oral Health Affect General Health?

Oral health is essential to general health. The mouth acts as a 'window' to the rest of the body, providing signals of general health disorders. A healthy mouth enables not only adequate nutrition, but also enhances social interaction and promotes self-esteem and feelings of wellbeing.

Poor oral health can have a significant impact on people's quality of life. It can also influence other diseases that they may be suffering. People with untreated oral diseases can experience severe pain, loss of sleep, inability to eat particular foods, loss of work or school and embarrassment about their appearance. These diseases can also accelerate the progression and severity of other illnesses.

The oral disease most frequently associated with medical conditions is periodontal disease. Though the biological interactions between oral conditions and other medical conditions are still not fully understood, it is clear that major chronic diseases share common risk factors with oral disease.

Your oral health might contribute to various diseases and conditions, including:

- Infective endocarditis (IE). IE is an infection of the inner lining of your heart (endocardium). Endocarditis typically occurs when bacteria from another part of your body, such as your mouth, spread through your bloodstream and attach to damaged areas in your heart.
- Cardiovascular disease. Heart disease, clogged arteries and stroke might be linked to the inflammation and infections caused by oral bacteria.
- Pregnancy and birth. Women with chronic periodontal disease are more likely to give birth to pre-term or low birth weight babies.

Additionally, certain conditions also might affect your oral health, including:

- Diabetes. Diabetes reduces the body's resistance to infection — putting the gums at risk. Gum disease is seen more frequently with greater severity among people who have diabetes.
- HIV/AIDS. Oral problems, such as painful mucosal lesions, are common in people suffering from HIV/AIDS.
- Digestive disorders. Recurrent mouth ulcers are occasionally a manifestation of coeliac disease and Crohn's disease.

- Osteoporosis. Bone and tooth loss in the lower jaw can be an early indicator of skeletal osteoporosis, which causes bones to become weak and brittle.
- Alzheimer's disease. Deteriorating oral health is seen as Alzheimer's disease progresses.

Other conditions that might be linked to oral health include eating disorders, rheumatoid arthritis, head and neck cancers, and Sjogren's syndrome – an immune system disorder that causes dry mouth. Because of these potential links, tell your dentist if you're taking any medications or have had any changes in your overall health, especially if you've had any recent illnesses or you have a chronic condition, such as diabetes.

The common risk factors that oral disease shares with other chronic diseases are:

Diet

A balanced diet provides the body with the appropriate quantity and quality of nutrients required to sustain health. Deficiency diseases such as anaemia result from the inadequate intake of specific essential nutrients. Overeating leads to obesity, a major health risk factor.

Tobacco Use

Tobacco contains chemicals that are harmful to the human body. Oral conditions caused by tobacco consumption include increased risk of periodontal disease, bad breath, discoloured teeth, an increased build-up of dental plaque, and delayed healing following periodontal treatment or oral surgery. Smoking is bad for the health: it increases the risk of several types of cancers, emphysema and other respiratory diseases, coronary heart disease, stroke, and diabetes. Smoking is also associated with adverse pregnancy outcomes, earlier menopause in women and sperm abnormalities and impotence in men.

Alcohol Consumption

Alcohol is a risk factor for cancer, cardiovascular disease, liver cirrhosis and trauma. Compared to non-drinkers, the risk of oral cancer is six times higher in those who drink alcohol.

Hygiene

Hygiene is a risk factor for periodontal disease and other bacterial and inflammatory conditions. Poor personal hygiene leads to inflammatory skin conditions and other bacterial infections.

Oral hygiene refers to individual habits and professional methods used to control the plaque that grows on tooth surfaces. If not removed regularly, dental plaque can lead to tooth decay and periodontal disease. Tooth brushing as a daily routine is the most important method of plaque control. Early assimilation of good oral hygiene into general hygiene practices promotes better overall oral health and general health. An association between poor oral hygiene and higher risk levels of cardiovascular disease, though the nature of the association is not yet understood.

Control & Stress

Stress and control are risk factors for periodontal disease and cardiovascular diseases. Stress is the body's reaction to external forces or events that cause physical or emotional tension. When a person feels stressed, adrenaline and stress hormones are released to prepare the body for the 'fight-or-flight' response.

While stress is a normal part of life, excessive stress can lead to health problems and lifestyle behavioural changes (e.g., taking up or increasing smoking, increasing alcohol intake, changing dietary habits, becoming physically inactive, neglecting oral and personal hygiene), which further increase health risks.

How individuals react to stress largely depends on their personality type. Even the most easy-going and adaptable people can suffer from stress if they lack a sense of control over aspects of their daily lives.

Chronic stress (e.g., low social support, low socioeconomic status, work stress, marital stress, caregiver strain) is a known risk factor for cardiovascular disease and periodontal disease.

Exercise and stress management techniques provide individuals with tools to cope with the anxieties in their lives. The most effective way to deal with stress is by correcting or modifying its underlying causes (e.g., low socio-economic status), however, this may be beyond the control of the individual.

Socio-Economic Status (SES)

The link between general health and SES is well established. In both high and lower income countries around the world, low SES is significantly associated with increased oral cancer risk, even after adjusting for potential behavioural factors. Thus, SES is an important risk factor: social disadvantage causes health disadvantage.

Fear of Dentist

Most people feel some level of anxiety before a visit to the dentist. But if your fear is stopping you visiting the dentist, it could be affecting your oral health.

It is important to visit your dentist regularly to ensure that your teeth, gums and mouth stay healthy.

So what can you do to help?
- Research – seek dentist recommendations from friends and family.
- Talk – Most dentists will be happy to openly discuss your fear and talk you through each step of a treatment.
- Support – Ask a friend to accompany you to your appointment.
- Signal – Agree on a hand signal with your dentist so you can indicate when you need a break during an appointment.

How Can I Protect My Oral Health?

To protect your oral health, practice good oral hygiene every day.

- Brush your teeth at least twice a day
- Floss daily
- Eat a healthy balanced diet and limit between-meal snacks
- Replace your toothbrush every three to four months or sooner, particularly if bristles begin to fray
- Attend regular dental check-ups
- Avoid tobacco use.

Contact your dentist as soon as an oral health problem arises. Taking good care of your oral health is an investment in your overall health.

naturopath

Your Body Knows Best

Julie O'Connell Seamer

*Could you view illness as an opportunity
for self-growth?*

*What if true health is only possible by embracing
the lessons our experience of sickness offer?*

I had my head inside our refrigerator one day, cleaning the shelves of various spilled liquids and old uneaten vegetable matter. This might seem a random and mundane event to share. However, while being so close to the inner workings of our modern day 'cold box', it struck me how the motor continues to run tirelessly, humming along loyally, without attention or recognition. This fridge has been part of my kitchen and world since pre-kids, so it has proven its worth. I thought to myself, what a blessing it is, that my family has cold fresh food which sustains our bodies, without having to do much apart from paying the power bill to run this fridge!

Have you ever thought about all the systems and mechanisms inside you in this way? Is it not a miracle that our hearts keep ticking, white blood cells engulfing pathogens, skin cells regenerating and lymph pumping against gravity, always? Why is it that we typically only rejoice at this gift when our good health is suddenly (or gradually) taken away?

Whenever I am sick I inevitably make inner deals with the 'devil' – or to whatever lurgy it is that is invading my organs, cheating me of wellbeing ... promising to honour my health fully this time; I will not forget to take my supplements or stay hydrated and rest when weary. I will be thankful for my amazing body, and not take it for granted. I will, I will!

Yet, predictably, as soon as I'm better again all those thoughts tend to fade and once more I am pushing harder than I should, eating on the run and taking on too many commitments. In my world time is money, and yet lack of time unfortunately usually equates to less conscious consideration of my body temple. So onward the cycle goes ... falling sick again, and wishing I had listened to myself, the little nagging symptoms or hints that things are starting to downward cycle, once more. Does this sound familiar?

Our Body Whispers Until It Has to Scream

Most of us mere mortals are quite skilled in ignoring such whispers. Even as a practicing naturopath, armed with a great deal of knowledge and readily accessible resources to rectify any underlying drivers to such 'whispers', I often find myself soldiering on. I don't deliberately set out to ignore the messenger, but most often I do find myself wishing away a health complaint, no matter how small it might be.

When we are in these situations, once our bodies are screaming in pain, or any other state of dysfunction, pharmaceuticals can bring a welcome quick fix. They allow a sense of temporary control, to be mistress of our body again, instead of at its whim. There's merit in this of course; we need to function after all. But when do these efforts become habitual? Are we shooting the messenger by shutting down symptoms that may be trying to disturb us for a deeper reason?

Sometimes things get the better of us. It might be tummy aches that become irritable bowel syndrome or it could be a sore joint that has never fully repaired after a childhood injury, and decades later it's still impacting our days. I broke a collarbone when I was a young horse-rider and it never fully repaired, from lack of care and attention. Because I know this is ultimately my own 'fault' I do try to avoid judging the 'seriousness' of issues like these with my patients in clinic. We all process stress, accidents, illness and dysfunction differently – things can be relative. At that time I wanted to prove myself strong to my father, and simply get back on the horse. Sometimes doing so isn't really honouring our greater needs, though.

In my naturopathic practice the common thread among all clients, male or female, young or older is the yearning to care for and acknowledge their individual needs while juggling family, work commitments, studies/education and other general pressures or goals pulling them in certain (sometimes conflicting) directions. Whether through mindset or physical actions, the one thing we can be sure of is that whatever paths we might travel, our bodies will tell us when we're 'out of kilter', and not listening to our inner callings. Typically we lean too far outward and fail to pause or truly take on board what our body tells us. Can you relate to this?

Listening to Our Body

It is important to acknowledge the subtle changes in our body. This seems common sense to me but the quick fix mentality of modern life (the general hectic pace with non-stop temptations to reach out and connect with everyone or anything via social media and the internet) doesn't often allow for much self 'checking in'. Naturally, when we stay disconnected, life and our body will usually bring us back inward – through illness, or a mild cause of disharmony – whatever it takes to interrupt or short-circuit our unhealthy ways!

Sometimes we must call the shots and draw a line in the sand too ... assessing what's true sickness and something constructed. This is an acquired skill – that necessary radar which alerts you when to push yourself and get out of a funk or rut, or to stop and listen. Often though, if our default is to go/don't stop, whether we experience a sudden or on-going loss of weight or a lump in our skin that persists, slowly but surely our body will call for our attention until we take note.

How often have you felt an impending virus or cold-sore building up within you, but you fail to deal with the situation, before it progresses? For most of us, life has become so multi-layered and all encompassing that we are completely unable to find space or time for rest, reflection and rejuvenation. Few of us could stop tending to our commitments and responsibilities to have a nap and try to sleep off a bug. So we become our own worst enemies, because meanwhile the body continues to present dysfunction or dis-ease if homeostasis isn't fully restored.

Even in my mid-40s now, I admit fully to still being an apprentice to my body.

Your Body is Your Teacher

When I was 27 years old I had been travelling solo around the globe, pushing my endurance and mindset to extremes. I'd hiked the Mt Annapurna range in the Himalayas, fueled by Mars bars and dhal bhat, surfed murky waters around Timor eating only rice, attempted being vegan while working as a horse riding instructor in America (which translated to a fries and drip coffee diet), having a wonderful time but not being mindful of what my body needed. I was active and yet my intake was poor.

Arriving back on home soil, a virus took hold of me and refused to subside. After weeks of being unable to hold anything inside my body (food and liquids) with increasingly debilitating lethargy, I woke one morning unable to feel my legs. The sensation of pins and needles alarmed me, as they weren't abating. After dragging my body across the road to our local beach, cold ocean water failed to remedy the numbness. I really started to panic. I couldn't walk! I was partially paralysed.

I was hospitalised with suspected Guillain-Barré Syndrome – a condition that can travel up the body. If it were to reach my lungs I could have died. To have instruments and syringes pushed into my legs with no feeling or response was extremely alarming. The news that I may never walk again sunk into my head like a lead weight. How could I possibly stay stationary? I felt I would go insane trapped inside an immobile body. And this was now only a month later!

The problem with this condition is that there was no specific line of treatment. After what felt like endless lumbar punctures, MRI scans, daily heparin shots in the stomach, rounds of medical students circling my bed to learn about this mysterious virus, I had not progressed. I was still unable to take myself to the toilet, stand up, dress, undress or work out how to fix this situation. Apart from finding ways to rebuild my defense system, there was little hope.

Whether it's cancer, a chronic illness or auto-immune disorder that you might experience – no matter the fact that others have walked your shoes, or been able to beat their disease, when it happens to YOU, life changes. Your perspective on what's important, the way you behave or go through your day … your relationships with people, and other parts of your existence somehow all change too. Even if it is simply that you no longer eat at the same cafes because your coeliac diagnosis has necessitated different ways of eating ... things aren't the same. An enforced self-review happens and certain internal shifts take place. And often these aren't so comfortable to ride through.

In my case, because my medical attendants were unable to provide solutions, I had to look for whatever I could find, that was not only within the realm of my own control but also somehow productive, even if that was one tiny step at a time.

For me, bed-bound, frustrated and suffering from the impact of hospital diet, lack of sunshine, fresh air and action, I had no choice but to dig deep. I wondered, *Was I honouring my functioning body previous to this?* Was I really grateful for my lack of sickness and energy, my capacity to push to extremes? Had I unconsciously been depleting my wellbeing to such an extent that somewhere, somehow, there was an aspect of this that I could turn around?

Your Body Hears Everything Your Mind Says

In my bed-ridden position, despite usually being quite pragmatic, I chose to believe that this was the case. This was spurred on while reading *The Tibetan Book of Living and Dying* by Sogyal Rinpoche. Perhaps a strange choice, but it felt like some part of me was passing on (if not dying!). The young reckless roaming Julie ... shifting into a more deliberate adult human being – while the doctors laughed at the seemingly drastic nature of this reading. I must admit, had I not been stuck there horizontally by the force of this virus, I may not have considered where I was actually heading in my life. What was I stepping toward? My legs were at a standstill and all I could ponder was my direction. Where was I planning to take them? Where was I going if I could will them back to mobility again?

I decided I had to start talking to my cells. Just like an Olympian visualising the success of their intended outcome, every day I literally willed my legs to work again, for my white blood cells to activate the necessary immune responses, and for this virus or issue to now leave my body. It was possibly a radical choice but I discharged myself from hospital and felt like a prisoner meeting the real world after an age of isolation. Everything sang to me – the sound of birds, the sight of clouds without a glass windowpane between us, even the humdrum noise of a rubbish truck collecting its load. Eventually my limp lower body responded – with a mixed regimen of herbal medicine, yoga and very intentional and regular meditation sessions, I pushed my way back to total wellbeing.

Sometimes Our Body Stops Us!

Although it was irritating to concede to this fact, I believe it is what happened for me. Many of us don't have the benefit of time to be able to ponder the underlying message of our symptoms. And of course it is often not needed. But sometimes, it is. Because if we don't, things can return to remind us of lessons not yet learnt. A case of glandular fever for instance, that never quite resolves, or childhood hayfever that can be overcome, but will surely continue to haunt you, if the underlying disharmony or deficiency is not addressed.

I was fortunate back then that I had no dependents and was able to fully focus on and dwell upon my situation, uninterrupted. It didn't happen overnight. There were many tearful days alone in my hospital bed, wishing I could be home or anywhere but there, followed by months of focused work on rebuilding my strength and mobility.

It was surely a challenging time but I learnt an important lesson: there is a fine line between managing symptoms and masking the real issues underlying your condition.

Are you resisting the messages your body is sending?

When we repeatedly shut off a pain message or any state of discord in our body/mind, are we ignoring the vital alerts our body is trying to express? Even when it's partially broken, we might automatically attempt to block any feedback our body sends us, refusing to allow our biology to become our biography. It is a fair call to take pain medications. It is a fair call to do what's needed to support our ability to get through the day ... providing at some point we do stop to consider what is happening, and why.

Back in hospital I did not want to identify as a partially paralysed or disabled person. I had determined to myself I would fight tooth and nail to get better and be back out running around like usual. So my only choice was surrender. And to listen. Everything that happens to us is a chance for reflection and learning. A chance to check in and recalibrate, as our very cells are doing at that given time.

From a wholistic viewpoint, our un-wellness often presents as polarity and disconnection. Although in our world of social media saturation we are supposed to be more connected than ever before, are we really connecting with ourselves as much as we ought to? My years in clinic have very clearly taught me this: it is vital to let our disturbances disturb us.

Symptoms arguably exist to correct imbalance. Any sickness represents an opportunity to delve further into or learn more about ourselves. Annette Noontil says in her book, *The Healing Power of Illness*, 'Symptoms can be seen as bodily expressions of psychological conflicts. They are able to reveal our current problems'. Without being too deep I am certain that any condition can offer a gift, if you are willing and receptive to take it.

To support your journey I would encourage seeing whatever health practitioner calls to you – be that a Physiotherapist, Masseur, Acupuncturist, your local GP, a Psychologist or whomever seems ready and able to help empower you in discovering the drivers to your symptoms. By addressing the underlying discord you will surely be more equipped in returning to good health and achieving your optimal longevity.

Remember too, it takes a village to raise a child, likewise for adults, it can take a village to support and maintain your ongoing wellbeing. As a Naturopath, I am always delighted and humbled to be part of others' journeys and efforts, in bringing a state of empowered wellness. No matter how healthy you are right now, if you begin to lose your sense of mortality or gratitude and respect for your body temple, rest assured your body will whisper, until it has to scream!

trichologist

Happy Health, Happy Hair

Megan Wright

'It is said that the eyes are the mirror to ones soul, I
believe that the hair is the mirror to ones health.'
– Megan Wright IAT

M y name is Megan Wright and I am a hair and scalp specialist, otherwise known as a trichologist. I have been practising for seven years with a previous history of hairdressing, as well as being involved within the hair and beauty industry – as an educator in both the private and public system – for the past 30 years. You might think that hair health has very little to do with body health, but from my experience it is a good indicator that there is more going on inside the body.

Trichology ... What is It?

Trichology is the scientific study of the hair and scalp. Trichology is a very specialised occupation and we are very privileged to assist patients with a vast number of differing hair and scalp concerns. Some of these concerns include, but are not limited to: various alopecias (hair loss) including genetic, hormonal, stress related, diffuse, unexplained sudden hair loss and patchy hair loss, to name a few. We also work with patients who have psoriasis; atopic dermatitis; ringworm and other fungal diseases and abnormalities of the scalp.

As a trichologist, I assess the patient's complaint with thorough consultation, incorporating the use of a magnifying apparatus called a Hair and

Scalp Polariser. This allows the user and patient to view the hair and scalp as a magnified image (60x, 100x, 150x).

Once an assessment has been made, we then create a treatment plan and/or course of action for the patient. I work with my patients holistically because I believe every facet of your life has a direct and indirect imprint on the health of your hair.

We recommend vitamin/mineral supplements; tinctures and topical creams, amino acids, and whenever appropriate, I work with my patients to implement the appropriate lifestyle changes required to maintain their hair and scalp health.

Throughout this chapter we will discuss the autoimmune deficiency and how lifestyle can have a direct effect on the health of your hair and scalp. We will discuss two particular hair and scalp disorders, their symptoms, how we can manage and treat them, and also prevention.

Autoimmune Diseases of the Hair and Scalp

I chose to share these two diseases with you because they both have similarities. We will discuss their symptoms, aetiologies and triggers, along with some treatments.

Psoriasis and Alopecia Areata

Psoriasis and alopecia areata are the two most common disorders that present in my clinic.

Both alopecia areata and psoriasis are autoimmune diseases, which are 'triggered' (for want of a better word) by some form of trauma, physical or emotional. The trigger may be different from person to person. Those who are not able to manage their stress levels etc. may be more likely to develop these symptoms.

Why are some people affected with psoriasis and alopecia areata and not others? What is the chance of you getting one of these disorders? If psoriasis and or alopecia areata are a hereditary disorder, then why can generations go without it becoming evident?

Facts:

- Both of these diseases can also be found on any area of a patient's body.
- Both alopecia areata and psoriasis are triggered by a trauma of some kind. A trauma could be: an immunisation, physical or emotional trauma, sudden weight loss, or any number of stressors.
- Both alopecia areata and Psoriasis are genetic disorders. This means that you and I may have the same amount of stress/trauma in our lives, but if I don't have the genetic predisposition for alopecia areata or psoriasis, it will not present that way.
- Neither psoriasis nor alopecia areata are contagious disorders.

Psoriasis

Psoriasis is a hereditary or genetic disorder. However, this does not mean that everyone will present with it. How a person manages their stress levels can have a great bearing on whether or not psoriasis becomes a part of their lives. It is not limited to the head. Psoriasis may present on any part of the body. The most common sites apart from the scalp are elbows, knees, arms and legs as well as fingernails.

Psoriasis appears to be flaky patches, which look silvery with an irritated redness underneath. Sometimes the area will be itchy and upon itching, the area may bleed easily.

Everybody manages their stressors differently. Unfortunately for some, the pre-disposition of psoriasis may be 'triggered'. A stress is anything unusual experienced by the body and can be experienced in times of fear, anxiety, excitement, physical and/or emotional trauma, even the death of a family member.

One of the body's ways of ridding the skin of the irritant is to provoke excessive scaling. This means that the skin cells in a particular area of the body replace themselves more rapidly. The cells are moving up to the epidermal layer much faster than usual. This is how the irritation and flakiness evolves with psoriasis. Normally, the skin replaces itself every 28 days or so, however, with psoriasis, the affected area is replacing itself much faster.

One Story:

I have a patient who visits me every six months to maintain her psoriasis management program. She began coming to me about one year after her husband had passed away and was complaining of an itchy, flaky scalp. Like most people, she had been to the doctor and tried all of the anti-dandruff products available on the chemist shelves, but nothing had worked.

After a thorough consultation and visual examination, we determined that her condition was in fact psoriasis and I then proceeded to develop a treatment plan, which was relevant and sustainable to her needs. She changed her home hair care products to vegan friendly, we incorporated amino acids and a vitamin-mineral supplement to her daily dietary input and she began a meditation program for that calming influence.

When she returned for her six-month check-in, there was a significant improvement in her overall scalp health. She still had a couple of little patches, which bothered her, but she was able to wear black clothing without looking like a 'ski slope'.

Treatments

Once your body has presented with psoriasis, there is no cure, however with a careful treatment plan and an ongoing maintenance program, relief may be found.

Some of the programs I recommend to my patients include the use of vegan friendly hair, scalp and cleansing products. This prevents animal by-products sitting on the skin and creating more 'food' for our healthy bacteria, and this limits the irritation.

Our scalp has millions of healthy bacteria living on its surface. When we have a condition such as psoriasis, our skin cells are reproducing at such a rate in some areas that we are unable to keep the excess skin cells from building up. Add into this mix, the thousands of hair strands, and it is very difficult to maintain a highly cleansed scalp. This is why there is irritation, redness and flakiness.

A vegan friendly conditioner has no animal fat (or animal by-products), therefore, we are not creating another food source for these healthy bacteria. This practice has made a notable difference in the treatment of my patients' symptoms.

Tar based creams and a thorough review of your dietary intake is also something to consider when treating psoriasis. I also take into consideration how you manage your stress levels. Do you have a regular 'time-out' session or even 10 minutes each day to find some peace and quiet, read a good book or sit and be still?

Corticosteroids and ultra-violet therapy are also recommended by medical practitioners and dermatologists.

Psoriasis is a condition that generally flares up every now and again and does not go away indefinitely once triggered. The way a person manages their stress levels, combined with the inclusion of a healthy diet with minimal processed foods, is most beneficial.

Quite often I get an influx of new patients in winter. This can be due to the climate changes, wearing hats, and sudden variables in temperatures etc.

If applicable and possible, swimming in salt water is a great relief for people with these symptoms.

Please note that the information presented here is a guide only. Please seek medical advice if you are suffering from any of these symptoms.

Alopecia Areata

The term Alopecia means 'hair loss'. Areata refers to the type, specific name or affected area of hair loss the patient presents. Like psoriasis, alopecia Areata is a genetic disorder. Again, this disorder does not necessarily present in every member of the family; it may even miss generations altogether.

As mentioned before, both of these disorders are 'triggered' by some sort of trauma or stress. Some triggers may include immunisations, emotional or physical trauma, viral or bacterial infection.

Alopecia areata presents as small round shiny hairless patches on the scalp. They may appear as small as a five cent piece and very often become larger if the trigger remains undetermined.

Alopecia areata is generally a self-correcting disorder, which means that once the 'trauma' or 'trigger' has been dealt with, the hair more often than not returns. Usually the first growth of hair is very fine white hair, but generally, the hair will thicken up and return to its original colour.

I always notify my patients that the problem may get worse before it gets better depending on how long ago the first patch was discovered.

A Story I'd Like to Share

One patient came to me with a couple of small patches of hair loss. I assessed her hair and scalp and decided her problem was, in fact, alopecia areata.

She was walking around the corner down the street when she 'bumped' into a man who had a pet snake wrapped around his neck! Bizarre, but true.

She told me that her entire body went cold and her heart felt as though it had stopped for a moment. A few months later she noticed the bald patches on her scalp and came to see me for advice. She said she had also seen a professor of dermatology and he had told her to get a wig and offered no other advice.

I assessed her scalp microscopically and found viable hair follicles, which indicated to me that there was still hope. If there is a follicle (hole for the hair to grow out) there was still a chance. We began her treatment regimen, which included amino acids, mineral supplements and a cleaner diet and the incorporation of some form of meditation or quiet relaxation (for healing time). I made sure she understood that her hair loss might get worse before it got better.

Upon her next visit, three months later, she wore a beanie. Oh dear, I thought ... yep, all of her hair had fallen out. So we reassessed the health of her scalp again and yes, I could still see healthy hair follicles all over her head. We continued with the treatment plan as expected.

Three months later she came back to me still wearing her beanie. I felt sad for her until ... tadaaa ... she whipped off the beanie and there was a healthy cover of hair! YAY! She has never looked back.

That is one of the happy ending stories. We found what the 'trigger' for her shock/trauma was and her body simply needed to recover and heal itself over time. There was every chance that her body could have recovered without the amino acids and mineral supplements, but I believe every little thing you can do to aid the recovery the better. This was an especially pleasurable success because she had been told by a professor of dermatology to 'never expect a healthy head of hair again and to invest in a wig.'

Not everyone has a story with a happy ending. I have another patient who has lost her hair and now wears a wig. She has lost eyebrows, lashes and all of her body hair. Mindset has a lot to do with it as does dealing with the 'trigger'. This particular patient's trigger was an emotional situation, which she found was very difficult to change. Once alopecia areata encompasses the whole body it is most likely going to become permanent and is therefore renamed alopecia universalis. This is most certainly not a regular occurrence.

That said, a very high percentage of my alopecia areata patients have had 100% hair growth return.

Now they must simply be aware that this is how their body deals with trauma and stress and keep a close eye on their stress management through healthy eating, meditation or deep relaxation and finding 10 minutes in each day to be still.

Treatments

Alopecia areata is generally a self-correcting disorder. What I mean by this is that usually over time, the hair loss recovers without much change. As we have spoken about also, is the 'What if it gets worse?' scenario. If the 'trigger' is not found, and the body is constantly being stressed, the symptoms – e.g. hair loss – will more than likely continue.

Depending on the condition, the inclusion of amino acids, multi-vitamins, minerals and a cleaner diet is all that a patient requires. Sometimes a psychologist may be suggested if the trauma is emotional. I always recommend some form of meditation or quiet relaxation. A lot of people find drawing or colouring beneficial.

There will be little to no change if the 'stress' is not changed.

As I stated with psoriasis, this information is a guide and from my experience. You must seek medical advice if you are suffering any of these symptoms.

Here are My Three Most Frequently Asked Questions ...

1. Will my hair ever grow back in those patches?

Alopecia areata is in most cases a 'self-correcting' disorder. What I mean by this is that once the body has suffered the initial shock or trauma, it generally begins to restore and repair the damaged area. If, however, the issue has not been resolved, or the body is not given enough opportunity to restore and repair, the disorder will most likely continue. Quite often when I see a patient, depending on their history, I make sure they are aware that the hair loss may often get worse before it gets better.

Once the trigger for your alopecia areata has been discovered and a treatment plan has been formulated, the recovery is generally very positive. I have only one patient who has suffered alopecia universalis (complete and permanent hair loss) and I believe the contributing factor to this outcome was the fact that they did not change the main stressor. Therefore, the body was never given the opportunity to begin the recovery process and the ongoing release of noradrenaline had a very detrimental effect in that patient's life.

2. Will alopecia areata or psoriasis come back?

The short answer to that question is yes.

When an autoimmune disorder such as AA or Psoriasis becomes physically active, it means that your body has been stressed or trying to get your attention for quite a while. These disorders, once they have become productive, will always have the potential to return whenever your immune system is run down and working hard.

However, the changes and improvements you make in your lifestyle and your ability to manage your external and internal stress levels, will definitely have an effect on the reoccurrence of either of these disorders.

3. Will psoriasis ever go away for good?

Like AA, once your body has suffered a 'trigger' you will always have the potential of a reoccurrence. Psoriasis is not curable. However, with the incorporation of proper diet, suitable home health care products such as vegan-friendly shampoos and conditioners, specific vitamin and mineral supplements as well as some form of relaxation for the healing process, psoriasis is very often treatable and with the right treatment program, often becomes a manageable condition.

Three actions the reader should take as a result of reading this chapter:

1. Be mindful of your stress levels if you know you have a genetic pre-disposition to either alopecia areata or psoriasis.

2. Go back to the basics in all aspects of your lifestyle. This includes cutting down on processed foods (eat raw, fresh, unprocessed produce); use vegan-friendly healthcare products, such as shampoo, conditioner and body cleansing products; drink 6–8 glasses of water each day.

3. Find at least one activity where you can absolutely stop and feel calm. I suggest meditation or meditative walking, even sitting in a your favourite cosy spot with a good book. You must allow yourself at least 10 minutes per day to stop and breathe.

These actions can be useful for general health regardless of whether you have these genetic predispositions. Hair, like nails and skin, will reflect how healthy you are on the inside. So if they are looking a bit dry, flaky, and patchy or off-colour, have a think about how well you are looking after yourself.

The Body as a Temple

Kylie Hennessy

'A yogi never forgets that health must begin with the body. Physical health is not a commodity to be bargained for, nor can it be swallowed in the form of drugs and pills. It is something that we must build up. You have to create within yourself the experience of beauty, liberation, and infinity. This is health.'

– B.K.S. Iyengar

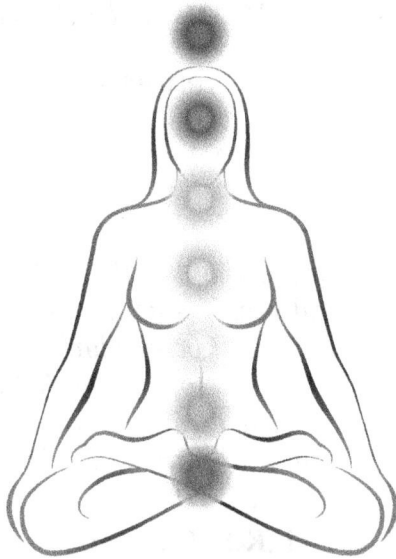

Crown Chakra		Spirituality
Third Eye Chakra		Awareness
Throat Chakra		Communication
Heart Chakra		Love, Healing
Solar Plexus Chakra		Wisdom, Power
Sacral Chakra		Sexuality, Creativity
Root Chakra		Basic Trust

When I began yoga I assumed it was simply a series of movements to make the body more flexible. I am not even sure the exact reasons I began to explore it, but what I fell in love with was that yoga is a great art, science and philosophy. Not only can yoga heal the body but also optimise its performance in all ways.

Even as a young girl I knew I wanted to be a doctor. I was always interested in how the body worked and how it healed. This led me to study a science degree in which I majored in biochemistry and chemistry. I loved and still love thinking about the body's complexities. Essentially, our body is almost an infinite amount of chemical reactions that are interconnected with our environment; but at the same time I wondered about emotions and the concept of a soul. I felt alone in my thoughts of this in a male dominated scientific world. Learning the details of chemical reactions that create, sustain, heal and balance a human body was mind blowing.

The ancient system of yoga is often referred to as an art and a science as it is a holistic system for creating health and wellbeing. It is both systematic and evidence based, as well as creative and transformational.

In terms of yoga, health is seen as not only as balance within the physical body but also the mental, emotional and spiritual bodies. These aspects of ourselves are interconnected and continuously influence one another. This is important to acknowledge when identifying how to use yoga to create a healthy body. Yoga as a practice encompasses postures (asana), breathing practices (pranayama), self observances (yamas and niyamas), meditation, visualisation and deep relaxation.

So What is Yoga?

Yoga, being a Sanskrit word, has various translations. It is derived from the root word for 'bridle' and is commonly translated to words such as: union, to yoke, and to join. Yoga does not just refer to a singular activity; it is a term that references a collection of practices.

We can think of yoga in its entirety as practices for *joining* the body, mind and breath, or bringing them back into synchronicity. We can also think of the practices as a way of *remembering and experiencing* that the body, mind, breath and spiritual self are unified and cannot be separated. Yoga is *a state*, a state in which we experience a sense of oneness and presence in the here and now. This is a very natural experience that many people encounter when in nature or in moments of love and connection with others. Yoga helps to access these moments and cultivate them more consciously from within, independent of external circumstances.

Yoga helps us develop a relationship with our whole self by bringing back alignment to our body, mind and breath, creating greater inner harmony and wellbeing as we move through life.

As Hippocrates once wrote, *'The natural healing force within each one of us is the greatest force in getting well.'* The modern day researcher Dr Herbert Benson has been at the forefront of producing the scientific evidence of this natural healing force. He has coined the term 'The Relaxation Response', the natural biological response, which activates this natural healing force. It has also been shown that many yogic postures, breathing techniques and meditation activate this healing response.

So Where Do I Begin with Yoga?

You begin yoga where you are. Many people feel they can't 'do' yoga because they are not flexible, they can't meditate because they can't sit still and their mind is too active. The practices of yoga are just that, a practice. The more we practice the easier things become.

It is often said, *'If you can breathe you can practice yoga'*. The benefits of yoga in improving our bodies' wellbeing are great.

Practicing yoga can improve:

- Flexibility
- Muscle strength and tone
- Alignment and posture
- Tension in the fascial system
- Proprioception
- Digestion and excretory system
- Body's detoxification ability
- Nervous system

- Hormonal or endocrine system
- Respiratory system and breathing quality
- Energy levels
- Sleep quality
- And more!

Patanjali's Ashtanga Yoga (8 Limbs of Yoga)

'Practice and all is coming…'
– Sri Pattabhi Jois

It is well known that Yogic traditions date back around 5000 years in India, making it one of the oldest sciences that exist today. It is widely accepted that one of the first written forms of the system of yoga was Patanjali's Yoga Sutras. Dated back to around 400 BC, it is this text that includes Ashtanga (8 limbs) Yoga. It is predominantly this text that modern yogis draw the wisdom and practices of yoga from today.

As the name suggests, it is not a ladder of hierarchy or sequential steps to follow, but limbs of a system that work together. These limbs are moral and ethical guidelines of how one might positively influence their own life. Many people find that they may begin with one limb, which flows through to other practices naturally, or they may find what they are looking for by predominantly adopting the practices of a few of the limbs.

The 8 Limbs

The 8 limbs are a guide or outline to discovering the benefits of yoga.

Yamas: Restraint

The Yamas are practices we can use in relating to the world around us, like moral codes and disciplines.

1. **Ahimsa:** Non-violence
   - Practicing non-violence towards ourselves and others. This includes being kind to our bodies, nourishing ourselves through good food, relaxation, and sleep etc.
   - Being kind to others and ourselves where possible.

2. **Satya:** Truthfulness
   - Being truthful to ourselves and others in turn helps to create a more relaxed mental and emotional state. We are valuing ourselves to say and follow our own truth in life.

3. **Asteya:** Non-stealing
   - This refers to non-stealing and not taking from others what is not yours.

4. **Brahmacharya:** Moderation in sexual behaviours
   - Practicing moderation in sexual activities through healthy relationships with ourselves and others.

5. **Aparigraha:** Non-possessiveness
    *   Trying to hold onto material things, people, or even ideas can cause us suffering by cluttering our mind and energy. Letting go of things is freeing and it helps us to grow and transform. Possessiveness can cause over-attachment, fear and anxiety.

Niyamas: Discipline

Niyamas refer to observances we can use within ourselves and self-disciplines.

1. **Shaucha:** Cleanliness
    *   Keeping cleanliness of our body and purity of thought. Simple practices of nourishing ourselves through cleaning and self care for our physical body. Maintaining cleanliness to areas like our skin, hair, teeth and fingernails and our surrounding environment can have a positive effect on our body's health.

2. **Santosha:** Contentment
    *   Cultivating an inner feeling of contentment and satisfaction. Observing and correcting thoughts and feelings of dissatisfaction towards things we cannot change or alter. It also relates to cultivating a feeling of contentment that is not related to external things or circumstances.

3. **Tapas:** Discipline
*   Commitment is required to continue with the practices in order to improve and maintain one's health. It is imperative to acknowledge Ahimsa (non-violence) when undertaking Tapas (discipline) in order to maintain a healthy relationship with your practices. It is a commitment practicing what is appropriate for you to create and maintain wellbeing

4. **Svādhyāya:** Self Study
*   To study oneself in the appropriate context for you. Perhaps through ancient wisdom texts, and/or modern psychological understanding, which might include the latest mind-body science. This helps us to increase our knowledge of human nature and positive states of health on all levels.

5. **Ishvarapranidhana:** Surrender to Divine or Higher Self
*   Having a belief in a greater power than our individual self, whether it may be nature, the universe, a form of God or a Divine. This helps brings peace and an ability to go with the flow of life. It reminds us we are a part of the whole however we may experience it.

Asana: Postures

Asana are postures in which we should be steady and comfortable, 'sthira sukham asanam'. The postures discipline the body to keep it disease free and preserve the vital energy or life force where possible. Steady and correct postures will also create steadiness and comfort in our physical body. This can aid meditation and prevent disturbances in the nervous system and mind.

Pranayama: Breath Control

These practices help to control our life force energies or prana. They can be used to calm, energise or bring balance. The breath is a very powerful way to bring all of our systems into balance. Significant physiological changes have been shown to occur with even simple breathing techniques – such as raising or lowering blood pressure, as well as releasing powerful pain relieving substances and feel good hormones such as endorphins from the brain.

Pratyahara: Withdrawal of Senses

Withdrawal of senses from their external objects, where we draw our attention to focus inside ourselves and use our inner senses.

The last three levels are called internal aids to yoga:

Dharana: Concentration

Concentration of the mind upon a physical object, such as a flame, the midpoint of the eyebrows, or the image of a deity.

Dhyana: Meditation

Steadfast meditation. Undisturbed flow of thought around the object of meditation. The act of meditation and the object of meditation remain distinct and separate.

Samadhi: Oneness

Oneness with the object of meditation. The experience is that there is no distinction between the act of meditation and the object of meditation – just a sense of oneness or being.

As you can see, the practices used within yoga are used to bring balance throughout our whole multidimensional system. Uniquely to yoga compared with other forms of exercise, the practices address tensions in our mind, our breath and/or our sense of self, all of which are seen to enhance our physical wellbeing.

It references subtle aspects to the human body (often referred to as our subtle bodies) such as our mind, emotion and breath. and how our physical body interacts with our subtle bodies. The health of our subtle bodies influences the wellbeing of our physical body, whilst our body's health influences our subtle bodies.

What Are The Subtle Bodies?

The Mind-Body Map of the Koshas

Referencing the aforementioned aspects that help derive health in yoga (mind, body, emotions and spiritual self), these aspects are known as our subtle bodies. Yoga has a variety of maps to describe the subtle bodies and their relationship with each other. One of these Maps is called The Pancha Maya Koshas – The 5 Illusionary Sheaths. *Maya* means illusion, veil or appearance so we can also think of the Koshas as the veils that encircle the True Self or *'Atman'*.

It is believed these sheaths conceal our true spiritual essence of inner peace, *Atman*. When there is disharmony within one of these subtle bodies, this inhibits the communication between them. When we remember and experience our true essence as peace, this too flows through the rest of our being.

The Five Koshas are:

1. Annamaya Kosha
- 'Anna' meaning food or Sheath of Food. Our physical body is ultimately made up of molecules from which are derived from the nutrients we receive through food.

2. Pranamaya Kosha
- 'Prana' meaning life-force that underlies our entire universe. It is the breath and the energy that flows throughout our system. The oxygen intake through our breath ultimately produces energy to fuel the functioning of our body. Through Quantum Scientific Theory we also know that molecules at their essence are fluctuations of energy. This energy is also referred to life force, our 'energy' body, chi or ki.

3. Manamaya Kosha
- 'Mana' meaning mind or Sheath of the Mind/emotions, mental/emotional Body. Science has now identified the molecules of emotions, which Dr Candice Pert describes as the *'connecting medium between mind and body, flowing between the two and influencing both'*.

4. Vijnanamaya Kosha
- 'Vijana' meaning knowing or Sheath of Wisdom, Wisdom Body or Inner Wisdom. It also relates to our ancestral wisdom.

5. Anandamaya Kosha
- 'Ananda' meaning bliss or Sheath of Bliss. Seen as divine understanding, love that is here/within and a blissful state that can be accessed within ourselves, independent of the external world.

Each Kosha is a different 'layer', which becomes subtler as we move toward our True Self. We can think of them as a representation of how our light shines through to our true self, which lies at the centre of our being. Disturbances can be sitting or begin in one effecting the others, which reduces our ability to feel/see our own light.

They are interconnected and inseparable.

With this map we can see that tensions or weakness in any one of these subtle bodies has a consequential affect on the others, jeopardising the state of our health. This is helpful in choosing appropriate yoga practices to create balance by identifying the possible layer, which the disharmony is arising from.

For example, low energy levels may be a result of poor breathing, which can be caused by anxiety. This in turn causes shallow breath and tension in the diaphragm muscle and physical tightness in chest.

Practicing Simple Yogic Breathing – also known as diaphragmatic breathing – can help to release such ailments. We could also combine this with some simple posture to enhance the breathing technique by releasing tension around the diaphragm, ribcage and back.

Another example is trauma in the Manomaykosha (emotional/mental trauma). This has the potential to cause either a dull or overactive mind (depression or anxiety) and will effect the flow of our life force or prana in the Pranamayakosha. This in turn will effect our physical body's (Annamayakosha) digestion, as well as create stiffness and pain in the muscles and fascial system.

We could use postures combined with yogic breathing to relieve the physical stiffness and pain by releasing the fascia, and muscle tension. This will improve alignment, allowing the energy to flow, promoting healing. This will further allow emotional healing to occur which will translate to improving digestion and reducing feelings of anxiety and depression. The practices also help people to develop the skill of mindfulness where they are focusing on the present moment. This has been proven to be an excellent aid for people living with chronic pain, whether it be emotional, physical or both.

The Mind-Body Map of the Chakras

Another map used within the Yogic system to describe our energy centres is that of The Chakras. The Chakras describe energy centres within our subtle bodily systems that are located along the spine, starting from the base up to the crown of the head. The Chakra System is one shared by many ancient cultures such as Tibetan Buddhism, Tantra and Hinduism. Although it can vary slightly, the basic understanding is that the Chakras are part of our subtle body system along with energy channels called Nadis or Meridians in Japanese Yoga and Traditional Chinese Medicine. The main channel of vertical energy, known as the Sushumna, consists of feminine, Ida, and masculine, Pingala, qualities. These energies also need to be in balance in our life for optimum health and wellbeing. The energy centres or Chakras, are meeting points along these energy channels and do in fact coincide with nerve plexus and endocrine glands which have a lot of energetic activity. Interestingly, the parts of the nervous systems and the endocrine activity in these areas relate to the qualities of these chakras that the ancient wisdom has described. We can think of each chakra as also consisting of each of the 5 Koshas of Sheaths as well as the written elements of the Chakras (as seen on page 128).

For example, disruption in the 4th or Heart Chakra can be caused by old emotions stored in the heart if they haven't been processed and released. This can lead to a lack of self-love and acceptance or an inability to give and receive love. This can create tension on a physical level, which can cause upper back pain and tightness. With some gentle breath work into the chest area, meditation as well as some postures, it can help to release the physical tension here. This then will aid in facilitating the emotions to be resolved, corresponding to a feeling of freedom and comfort in the chest and upper back. This allows the Heart Chakra to flow and experiences of unconditional love and compassion to naturally arise. Giving and receiving love becomes easier.

Another example is pain in the base of the spine and hips relating to chronic fear and feeling of insecurity. Using postures to realign this area, develop strength and find a sense of grounding can help to find similar alignment on a mental/emotional level too. Most basic standing postures Tadasana or mountain pose are wonderful for this. This rebalances the Base or Base Chakra, restoring a sense of security and alleviating misalignment and pain in this area.

Where and How to Learn Yoga?

As a part of your yoga journey, remember to practice Satya, listening to your truth. You may try several teachers and styles over the years. As your life changes it is beneficial to acknowledge and apply your practice accordingly to support and maintain your wellbeing. This can change depending on stages of life and/or particular life circumstances that effect where, when and how you can practice.

Be kind to yourself and remember there are many practices to yoga. As they say. 'If you can breathe you can practice yoga'. Certain modifications or guidance may be required to find the practices and support you need to begin yoga and continue your journey to creating and maintaining a healthy body.

Teachers are there to guide you, to help direct you to listen to your truth, inner wisdom and body's wisdom for health and wellbeing. Yoga is a pathway to discovering yourself and what health and wellbeing means to you and for you. You may need to try a few classes and teachers until you find what is right for you. Tell the teachers what you are looking for and they can help you find what you need.

'The master functions as a friend. He holds your hand and takes you on the right path, helps you to open your eyes, helps you to be capable of transcending the mind. That's when your third eye opens, when you start looking inwards. Once you are looking inwards, the master's work is finished. Now it is up to you.'
– Osho – The Zen Manifesto #1, 1989

Remember practice makes perfect. Permanent changes happen over time and with practice. Sometimes change happens quickly and sometimes slowly and that is perfectly OK. The change that yoga will bring to you will be different to what it brings your neighbour; it will produce the changes you wish to see for yourself. Yoga brings balance throughout the subtle bodies and the physical body. There are many pathways and it begins with the first step, and as said by Ashtanga Yoga Teacher Eileen Hall, *'Get in a position to change your life'*. Yoga isn't just a practice for fitness; it is a practice of life.

Yoga helps me live a full life, which within all the complexities of being a mum, a small business owner and a full time yoga teacher and yoga therapist. I can return to an inner deep peace and infinite resource of love always. It feels very cliché to say it but it is a discovery of the self, a self-discovery that changed my life forever.

Verse 42 of The Narada Bhakti Yoga Sutras

tadeva sadhyatam tadeva sadhyatam

tat – that (grace)
eva – alone
sadhyatam – cultivate.

Cultivate grace alone, cultivate grace alone.

The Metaphysical World
– The Body Never Lies!

Anthony Kilner

The human body is an amazing instrument – a sophisticated, multifaceted network of systems that collaborate to ensure life from the moment of inception to the time of death. Its functions are so intricate that medical science is continuously making new discoveries.

Eastern and Western medicine offer diverse and often contrasting perspectives on how to achieve a healthy body. Dieticians and chefs try to educate us on how to combine food groups to assist the body to achieve optimal health. Drug companies spend millions of dollars, constantly looking for ways to help people achieve a healthier lifestyle. All of these methods have merit. My approach is to find the right balance.

As a Psychic Medium and a person who facilitates Vibrational Energy Healing, I understand that there is another world that is often forgotten or ignored when it comes to having a healthy body – the Metaphysical World.

Metaphysics is a branch of philosophy that looks at primal causes and first principles such as being, what we are, who we are, and why we are here – the fundamental nature of us as a 'being' in time and space, and how we as humans understand the world around us.

Most people, at some point, wonder about their existence. What is the purpose of their lives? Every person I know has wondered how life works, what has made the universe and why? Cause and effect is another big question that people wonder about, topping the list with, *What happens when I die?*

This is one reason our historians are so important – they compile all of our great philosophers, writers, poets and songwriters' works, in conjunction with their emotions and stories, to record our history and ultimately our evolution. This information is then available to help us try to understand what makes us who we are and how everything metaphysical connects with science and medicine. This is where worlds collide.

There is a lot more to metaphysics, however in terms of what I am covering in this chapter we are looking at the body as an organism that speaks to us through its sub-conscious actions as well as through its conscious ones such as pain.

Reading this chapter may challenge your belief systems and possibly your religion. I am not trying to change people's beliefs. I am offering something else to consider – a different perspective on life that may help you, or others around you, to get a glimpse of one possible interpretation of the world we live in.

We are conditioned from birth to believe many things, some of which may not be true. To gain a healthy body, readers will need to confront their own scepticism. True scepticism is about listening, trying to comprehend and then disbelieving or perhaps accepting that something cannot be explained properly – just yet!

We are not simple beings – we are a spirit having a human experience. Part of that experience is dealing with the human body with all of its beauty and flaws, and what that entails. Part of the reason we are here is directly related to the human body and all of its faculties.

As an energy source alone, we cannot experience what it is to be human. Without a physical body we cannot fully appreciate what it is to touch other humans, animals, plants and the Earth itself. We wouldn't know the incredible, life-changing emotion felt by parents touching their newborn child for the first time or that first passionate kiss that leads to the first intimate contact with a partner.

Our other physical senses also come into play with the amazing textures this physical world has to offer – the ability to smell life, the ability to hear sounds that create emotions within us, and the taste of good wine and food to name just a few things. These are our exclusive human traits and gifts that define who we are on this planet.

The downside to this, of course, is that we are born to die. In our human form we are subject to internal dis-ease as a result of our specific DNA and external dis-ease from factors such as UV exposure, chemicals, foods and many others, all of which contribute to our eventual death. Metaphysics adds another dimension to this with the addition of the mind as a controlling factor over our body. What the mind believes the body understands, and what the mind controls the body does. Our mind controls so much of what the body does, from the release of chemicals that influence emotions and physical responses, to electric impulses that drive the body's mechanics. The brain regulates on a physical level what the mind reacts to externally.

In the first book of the *Health Conscious Series*, how to create a healthy mind was explored in detail. Achieving a healthy mindset is imperative to creating a healthy body. But how does one create a healthy body? The answer is almost too simple – we listen to it!

The body is a well-tuned organ that will respond to everything we do to it. We are all guilty of ignoring it though, when it is telling us something is wrong, and we ignore some signs more so than others. We are not as good at listening to the language of the body when it is internal.

If you are riding a motorbike through the scrub and have an accident, your body will register any pain by signalling the brain. The brain then lets us know where that pain is and we generally deal with it appropriately. We also take the message on board for future reference. The expression, learning from our mistakes, is our body and brain trying to avoid that pain again.

If the body on the other hand, says there is pain or discomfort internally, many of us ignore these signals or use painkillers or drugs to try to mask the pain. It is only when the pain becomes unbearable we finally visit a doctor. Often, by this stage, the prognosis is shocking and we discover that our body is dying – we ignored the signs to our detriment.

From birth we begin to learn what our limits

are and yet we continually push those limits until we break down. Imagine being perfectly in tune with your body, enabling you to live a long and happy life.

The more we understand and listen to our body the easier it is to recognise the signs telling us there is something wrong or out of whack. Failure to identify these signs can allow problems to turn into serious issues. Both the success and failure of this communication comes down to how our mind works.

Our mind or our brain tells us whether or not we are okay, but it also allows for addictions that kill our physical body, it dictates what chemicals, such as adrenaline, serotonin or endorphins, are released into the body to deal with dis-ease and pain and it is easily impacted by external stimuli such as drugs or human behaviour that can raise us up or crush us.

Eastern and western doctors, healers, psychiatrists, counsellors, kinesiologists and therapists of all descriptions around the globe, are starting to realise that people who live with constant anger and negativity can create an unhealthy body, leading to major internal dis-ease. While on the flip side, people are living longer, happier lives by being positive in their thought processes.

Thought processes, conditioning and beliefs, can play a huge part in whether a person is pre-disposed to being negative or positive – the old adage of a glass half full versus a glass half empty.

The best way a person can heal their body is with their mind – being proactive and positive.

This understanding alone has started to blossom in my lifetime around a very connected world medically, scientifically, and spiritually. This is the holistic approach I take with my clients with mediumship and energy work.

The key to a healthy body is to understand the signs the body gives and work out ways to interpret and then deal with them. I am not a doctor or medically trained other than with First Aid. I base my understanding on over fifteen years working with real people in real situations with real results, some positive and some not.

In my world, the body tells us what we need to know both objectively and subjectively. Objectively is external to the mind, factual, the actual physical feeling of your body. Subjectively is of the mind, metaphysical and requiring interpretation. Both of these understandings can be combined to offer a holistic awareness of the body.

As an empath, when I do readings or energy work, I quite often feel pain on my body which relates to the client. I will start the conversation along the lines of, 'I am not a doctor, but I am experiencing this pain here and this pain there.' I would then ask the client if they understand the pain that I have described. This is objective pain.

I would then go on to give them a subjective meaning for that pain as well. For example, pain in the shoulders might indicate they are carrying a heavy burden. The pain is a trigger to guide me into a specific area of that person's life.

Objective pain in an area of the body is real pain and there will be a specific medical reason for that pain. For example, you have pain and swelling in both your knee joints, more so on the right side than the left that is there when walking, standing still or sitting. The medical reason for the pain might be osteoarthritis. However, before we deal with that pain, with drugs or with other more natural methods, let's consider the subjective understanding.

The knees represent flexibility and ego in a person's direction. The smoother the joints are, the more fluidity is achieved, pain free, in that direction. The swelling indicates fluid retention. Fluid retention represents moisture – fluid and water – representing emotions. Subjectively this would mean retained emotions in a person's direction and possibly about the ego ruling the mind.

The left leg represents the past and the right leg the future. In our scenario the right leg is worse than the left. This could mean that the person has been through a lot of emotional turmoil in their life and while they think that they have understood and moved on from it, there might be some residual emotions that still need to be dealt with. The right knee represents the emotional turmoil the person is still going through as they attempt to move forward in life. This might represent choices – work choices, family choices, relationship choices – needing to be made that are emotional or even confronting ideology and being able to change their mind about the way they perceive the world.

There could also be an aspect of ego or self-righteousness in sore knees, e.g., *I am not going to bend down to someone I don't respect or love as I see myself as better than them.* This is the person with the pain's issue and might reflect their emotional inability to heal themselves.

I believe that an open and honest discussion with this person could change their circumstances for the better. Over the years I have found that when you discuss personal issues with people they can often be stoic in their responses, which means they are denying on some level what has happened with them emotionally. That stoicness means they never accepted the truth of how they feel on any level and therefore they will never feel totally happy within themselves.

Another way to understand how this metaphysical or subjective stuff works is to understand that in life we can suffer bullying, shame, grief, anxiety, despair, love, heartbreak and trauma. Some of us can just seem to put these experiences aside and move on, for others it can consume their lives, while some manage to function in a limited way yet are never happy with who they truly are.

Attaining a greater understanding of the way the metaphysical world operates, offers a way to move forward into a new life. This new awareness allows us to love ourselves – that is our mind, body and spirit as a whole unit, which, in turn, will help us to navigate through our existence and journey on this planet!

Now for the juicy bits!

Listen to your body. When your body communicates pain or a problem in a certain area a subjective interpretation can help you resolve the core issue. Below is a basic list of body parts and aspects of self that they represent subjectively.

This list is a guide only with the aim to get you started understanding what physical pain and ailments can represent. Don't forget men and women are different in parts of their body structure so interpretation of those areas needs to take this into account.

If you are experiencing pain I suggest you deal with it on multiple levels to give yourself the best chance of being pain free and happy. Don't be a martyr with pain or ignore your body's signals, as it could be detrimental to your health. Whether it's eastern, western or spiritual healing, find what works for you and deal with it.

Body Part	What they represent
Hair	Ego, life's changes and experiences.
Head/Face	What we show to the world, aspects of ego.
Eyes	Ability to see into all aspects of past, present and the future.
Mouth	Ability to show and express sensitivity.
Nose	Ability to breathe calmly and distinction in all aspects of life. The ability to recognise one's self.

Teeth	Ability to help nourish one's self and make decisions – chewing over things.
Ears	Ability to hear one's self, spirit or others.
Brain	The body's computer. The ability to process information from multiple sources internally or externally.
Bones	Structure in life.
Neck	Ability to see where you have come from and where you are going.
Back	Support in life.
Shoulders	The ability to carry burdens. Many people carry stress in the shoulders.
Upper Back	Feelings of betrayal.
Middle Back	Guilt, carrying past burdens.
Lower Back	Financial concerns, lack of financial support.
Hips	Mother or mothering issues. The link between balance in all things.
Arms	The ability to carry life's experiences.
Wrists	Flexibility in grasping life's challenges.
Hands	Strength to grasp life and its experiences.
Left Hand	Past, male aspects.

Right Hand	Future, feminine aspects.
Little Finger	Children, family
Ring Finger	Relationships, good and bad.
Middle finger	Sexuality and anger.
Index Finger	Dominance, will and ego.
Thumb	Under the thumb, worry and self-belief
Stomach	Ability to digest life, nourishment.
Bowels	Ability to let go of waste in life.
Heart	Love and the ability to pump or operate in life, the centre of your being.
Blood	Life force, joy in life's flow
Legs	Strength in direction
Knees	Stability and flexibility
Ankles	Flexibility in direction, guilt or inflexibility
Feet	Stability and flexibility in direction and the ability to change direction. Left, right, backwards and forwards, on tippy toes to see further.

In addition to interpreting messages from the physical body, there are also emotional issues that trigger physical conditions. Subjective interpretation of these may help lead a person to better understanding themselves and their health.

Listed on the following pages are some basic human emotional and physical problems and the connection they may have with metaphysical manifestations. Many of these conditions are the result of negative thought processes.

There is not enough space to provide a lot of detail here so these are just some of the basics. The subject matter below is a combination of works I have studied/researched and personal experience and is by no means definitive. Readers may like to explore the book references below for more detail.

Addictions

Having spoken to and worked with many people with addictions, one of the common themes is their lack of self-love. This person will often run from and not be able to face their fear, instead using escapism as a way forward. These people often struggle to forgive themselves and the body responds with sadness, emotional distress and can't deal with responsibility properly.

Anxiety

Anxiety has a list as long as you can imagine and is often caused by self-belief issues, fears and guilt, with the body not able to cope or trust in the flow of life. Internally, this can lead to stomach issues, along with possible blood pressure problems.

Cancer

Many cancers are caused by deep-seated hurt, anger or guilt that is eating away at the mind and body. Depending on where the cancer is in the body, it will highlight which feelings are being repressed and need addressing, e.g. bowel cancer could be related to anger problems that have never been let go.

An interesting thing about cancers is that many people can carry the gene in their DNA for a specific cancer, yet it doesn't manifest in the body of one person while another can die from it. This is a result of external factors and emotional differences that have triggered the cancer to start growing. There have been papers written on this subject that can be researched online and genetic DNA predisposition testing is becoming more and more popular for people trying to achieve a healthier body and longer life.

Depression

Depression is such a huge issue and can be caused by so many factors (both internal and external) that it can be a hard dis-ease to understand and work with. Feelings of hopelessness, sadness, unworthiness, anger and frustration can manifest physically as depression, the body going into shutdown mode, and possibly leading to eating disorders and many other physical ailments.

Fear

Fear is a debilitating emotion that can cause stomach issues as we either cramp up and hold tight or at the other extreme we release everything. The body in fight or flight mode will often expel unwanted excrement in order to run faster or be stronger to fight with. Fear can also lead to adrenal fatigue from being in a constant state of anxiety. Lungs and breathing can often be affected by fear as well.

Guilt

Guilt is a perplexing thought process that can affect the body in more ways than one. We often feel guilty for the simplest of reasons – forgetting to say goodbye to a person, the choices we've made, or possibly something more extreme such as committing a crime.

Guilt can lead to self-loathing, depression, anxiety, anger and addiction scenarios, which in turn can lead to stomach issues, weight loss and more.

In understanding guilt, we need to forgive ourselves because we can't change the choices we have made. We need to make new choices to release the guilt and love ourselves again.

Overweight

Often people carry weight for various reasons, from the body malfunctioning physically to low self-esteem. When discussing who they are as a person, it often comes out with overweight people that they are oversensitive and feel the need for protection or to offer protection. Being oversensitive to life's challenges can manifest as anger and the struggle to forgive or accept forgiveness.

Resentment

Anger is normally the first response by someone being rejected. With time and nourishment that anger feeds on itself, causing stomach issues. Anger is a volatile emotion that the body responds poorly to.

Tears

As a boy I was taught not to cry, not to express my emotions, which in turn lead to not really understanding the emotional flow of life. Girls are allowed to, or expected to cry, which is why in many cases they are better at expressing themselves emotionally than boys. Blocking emotions means the body holds onto fluids and can never be as fluid in life as it could be.

Worthiness

Worthiness ties in with self-belief. How many times are we put down by our peers, bullied by other people who are struggling with their own lives and, in many cases, hiding behind bravado and hurting others?

The emotional responses to dealing with this issue can be strong, which leads to the body struggling to deal with emotional issues around them. This can result in tension in the body caused by frustration and, again, anger is one extreme reaction while timidity and shyness can be at the other end. Timidity can also lead to anxiety and associated eating disorders.

When you understand what the body is saying it becomes easier to look holistically at the message and delve into more detail about the situations you are experiencing. The hard part is working out a way to change your life accordingly so that you can move forward. Making these changes will require some thought and effort on your behalf.

The Challenge to Your Beliefs

Am I willing to change? Can I change? Am I remaining this way because I believe I am right and therefore feel I do not need to change?

In order to really understand what our body is saying to us it might help to look at things around us from a different and maybe new perspective. One point to consider is past lives, future lives and how Quantum Consciousness flows into the picture.

The theory of Quantum Consciousness embraces science and philosophy in a broad way and, of course, ties in with Quantum Physics. Quantum Consciousness explores the possibility of parallel timelines within lives.

Many people believe in reincarnation and that past lives are linear in the way that they work. This means that you leave one life for another and through time you accumulate lives like shoes. Many shoes to walk many paths!

During each life we attract good and bad karma and we have specific lessons to learn based on this karma and the experiences we set ourselves up for in the next life. Following this theory, ailments in our bodies, thought processes and actions from a previous life can impact us in our current life.

This theory can be evidenced by the fears we have. Some people may have a fear of drowning, or perhaps enclosed spaces. In a past life, this person may have drowned or been trapped in a mineshaft. There would then be an explanation for the fear they now feel. Having this explanation provides an understanding that can be used to find a solution to overcome such fears. This information can be discovered through past life regression. Past life regression is a natural therapy that takes people on a journey into their previous lives to uncover reasons for their current life issues.

Through my work doing past life regression, I have encountered situations such as this. In one case I established that at roughly the same age in a previous life, my client had drowned, and thus had developed a fear of water at that age in this life. By working through how the drowning occurred and the karmic ramifications, the person was then able to get back into the water.

In many cases the physical body is affected by past life issues. This is a fairly complicated topic, which needs more time to explore fully. Quantum Consciousness is also another discipline that considers the effect of multiple lives.

In Quantum Consciousness we gain an understanding that all our lives are running concurrently, much like Neo in *The Matrix Reloaded* when he walks into the control room to meet the Architect and there is a wall of TVs all showing him living different lives in different times yet somehow it's all linked together. For anyone that hasn't seen *The Matrix*, it's worth a watch as it covers some trippy thoughts on life, as we know it!

Like a past-life regression, practicing Quantum Consciousness relies on meditation and/or a form of hypnosis to calm the mind of the client and allow them to enter into every aspect of this life from a child to an elderly state and look both backward and forward in the current life. From here there is a process to go into each life (past, present or future) and from there, gain an understanding of what occurred in that life. At this point, it is possible to group all the lives that have suffered from the same issue and work through that issue to heal it in those lives, as well as in the life you are leading now.

This is pretty trippy and yet when I heard about it for the first time it made sense. The ability to heal the body and mind in this here and now life then becomes easier to achieve. Knowing that it's healing the parts of your concurrent lives as well is mind-blowing.

Quantum Consciousness links the parts of our soul that reside in our physical bodies in each life through our Soul Collective. Our Soul Collective or Over Soul, is the spiritual consciousness of all our lives held as an energetic source in the spirit world. If this theory can be grasped then it makes it easy to come to terms with the fact that we have access to every life, and that life's experiences, through our soul connection.

Through that soul connection we can find our truth and purpose in life, which means we can heal ourselves of many of the dis-eases we experience in this life. I did mention earlier both these past and concurrent life theories can, and will, challenge your belief processes!

There is a wealth of more detailed information available on these theories on the net and in books. I have listed some books that can get your feet moving in a direction that could help clear your mind and help you live a long and happy life.

Help and Support

Coming to an understanding of the metaphysical world, of subjective and objective information and Quantum Consciousness, is not easy. There are books, workshops, and esoteric means of learning many of these theories and I would suggest taking time (time is love) to discover how each theory sits with you. Putting this learning into practice will require changes in your thought processes that could lead to massive changes in your life and the lives of those around you. Keep in mind change means making choices and the best choices are informed and open minded ones.

Meditation is a great starting point. Allowing your consciousness to drift into the dis-ease to try and heal it could potentially change your life. Learning meditation will give you and your body the ability to relax, sleep, heal and function to its best ability.

Affirmations are another positive tool, like prayers and self-belief, which can improve a person's health. Saying an affirmation three times a day, writing it down and leaving it where you can read and see it will help you to believe it!

Here are some examples – one verse for Mind, Body and Spirit and it can be modified to suit any affirmation required.

I am open to the universe to receive perfect health.

I am open to the universe to receive perfect health.

I am open to the universe to receive perfect health.

I am open to the universe to realise self-love within my whole being.

I am open to the universe to realise self-love within my whole being.

I am open to the universe to realise self-love within my whole being.

I allow myself to be open and honest from my heart to be loved.

I allow myself to be open and honest from my heart to be loved.

I allow myself to be open and honest from my heart to be loved.

When I see myself, I see my soul and its place in a universe of infinite love.

When I see myself, I see my soul and its place in a universe of infinite love.

When I see myself, I see my soul and its place in a universe of infinite love.

I give myself permission to be happy, healthy and whole.

I give myself permission to be happy, healthy and whole.

I give myself permission to be happy, healthy and whole.

References

Louise Hay – You Can Heal Your Life

Annette Noontil – The Body is the Barometer of the Soul

Peter Smith – Quantum Consciousness, Expanding Your Personal Universe

Brian L Weiss – Many Lives Many Masters

Anthony Kilner – Practical Mediumship – A Guide to Understanding Psychics, Mediums, Dreams and Physical and Metaphysical Information.

publisher

Is Writing Bad for You?

Blaise van Hecke

It's hard to remember when we didn't have computers. When I was studying HSC (now VCE) back in the 80s I felt very lucky to have a little portable typewriter to put together my stories and essays. Most likely, sitting at a typewriter was equally as bad as it is to sit at a computer, but there weren't all the other things to do on a typewriter like check emails, go online to social media or troll the internet. This meant less time hunched over the keyboard. If you needed to look up the spelling of a word, you got up to look for the dictionary rather than go onto Google for an online dictionary.

When you're in the zone, it's easy to lose track of time as you tap away at your computer keys. Before you know it you've been bent over your desk for hours, wondering why you have a headache, sore neck or backache. There's no doubt that the technological age isn't good for our bodies because of these long periods of sitting at the desk, our posture deteriorating as the day wears on.

You would think that writing was a fairly low risk activity but, in actual fact, there is a need to make sure that you look after your body. There are a number of health risks associated with writing, such as chronic neck and back pain, constant headaches and, in the extreme, digestive problems. By making adjustments to your physical space, ensuring plenty of physical activity and eating well, the 'danger' of computer life can be alleviated.

Workspace is Important

Like any physical activity, when you do it for a prolonged period of time, your body will seize up or suffer from inactivity or repetitive actions, such as RSI (Repetitive Stress Injury). For this reason you need to design a workspace for your body and the work that you're doing. From a writer's point of view (or office work in general) you need to look at how many hours on average you spend at the desk. If all of your work involves you sitting at the desk all day working on the keyboard, you need to find ways to break this up. Your body will not like being sedentary for seven hours a day.

I have heard that sitting at the computer all day is as bad as smoking. That's a pretty broad statement and has varying degrees of impact on your body because a pack-a-day smoker will do more harm to their body than a social smoker who might just have one or two cigarettes a day, just like sitting for ten hours a day will be different to three hours. The point of this is that people don't take notice of the impact of a sedentary lifestyle and how harmful it is to their health.

This is where you need to listen to your body. Tune into it. Set your workspace up for optimum efficiency and to look after your posture. If you need to get a physical therapist to assist with this then do so. It's worth the money. If you say 'I can't afford it', ask yourself, 'Can you afford to be sick?' Because if you don't make these adjustments to your physical needs you will get sick. You'll spend more money on chiropractors and physiotherapists later on and you'll feel years older than you really are. And just because you don't have any issues now, wait a few years – they'll start cropping up and you'll feel like everything snuck up on you.

The most basic adjustments to your workstation can improve your situation. So here are some questions to ask yourself:

1. Have you got a decent office chair?
Your chair should be adjustable for both height and tilt. This is because everyone is different in height and most office desks are a standard height. If you're 165 centimetres, you will need your chair higher than someone who is 178 centimetres.

2. Do you have a footrest?
This is also related to height. If you're shorter than average, you need a footrest to make up for the chair set at a higher level.

3. Does your space have good lighting?
Looking at a computer screen all day can tire your eyes. Make sure the screen isn't too bright, or too dull, and that the room lighting works in conjunction with what you work on. Sometimes you may need to increase the size of your viewing panes, or the text to help. Or maybe you need to get your eyes checked to make sure you aren't overexerting them.

4. Is the computer at the right height?

This is relative to the chair to desk ratios and is important so that you're not tilting your head too high or low and thus causing issues with your neck.

5. Is heating and ventilation adequate?

This might sound very basic but so many offices are not healthy in this respect. Too hot and you get sleepy; too cold and you start shivering and tense your muscles.

6. Does the feng shui work for you?

This might sound a bit outlandish but sometimes reorganising your space can make you more productive. It can be what might seem insignificant like having your back to the rest of the office, or being able to look at nice scenery. There are many things that can help you feel more positive and happy in your environment. Maybe even a shiny green plant on your desk, or a favourite photo of a family member.

7. Are there distractions?

This is not so much a health issue but more a productivity issue. If you are a good procrastinator, like many writers, you need to remove distractions where possible so that you can get down to the writing and not spend longer than necessary at the keyboard.

8. Are you working on a laptop or desktop computer?

You may think there is no difference with these but a desktop computer is much easier to adjust to suit your physical needs because the screen and keyboard are separate. Because a laptop has an inbuilt keyboard, you are having to make different adjustments to your body. Quite often the laptop will cause you to tilt forward more and crane your neck at a more dramatic angle than is good for you. Working at a laptop for long periods is very bad for your posture and should be avoided especially as many people will sit on the couch with it on their lap. When possible, it's a good idea to set your laptop higher than your lap and to use a separate keyboard. This is not always practical as the idea of a laptop is its portability.

All of these questions may seem trivial but small adjustments can improve your posture and prevent chronic physical issues in the future.

Movement is Vital

Once you have your physical space set, don't think that everything is taken care of and you'll be able to sit at the computer for hours. Variety and movement are vital for physical health and wellbeing. Humans are meant to move. We have hundreds of muscles and bones that allow us to do this so sitting in one position for a long time will cause problems. Again, tune in to your body.

Close your eyes for a moment and tune in to your heart beat. It never stops while you are alive. It's pumping blood around your body, delivering vital nutrients to where they are needed. Keeping you alive. And there are other systems in your body doing equally important tasks. Basic biology classes in high school taught me that movement helps all these systems work at their best. Movement creates all kinds of things like heat and oxygen that help these systems flow better, which in turn improves our immunity (aside from other things).

Close your eyes again and tune in to other parts of your body. What is your posture like right now? I bet you straightened up a little at that question. If you are slumped a bit, think about the organs in the lower part of your body. Are they possibly squished up? Do you sit a certain way so that your neck, shoulders, or lower back feel at an angle or tight?

For the next few days, take note of your posture and how often you change your position. When you do change your position, what do you do? Do you get up and move about?

Here are some actions to take to help you to move more often:

1. Set a time to get up from your desk to get a drink of water. This could be every 30–40 minutes.

2. If possible integrate other tasks throughout the day that make you move. These could be filing papers, talking on the phone (stand up while you're talking), taking out rubbish, making a cup of tea.

3. Aim to get up and walk around the room a few times each day. Better yet, take a short walk outside if possible for 10–15 minutes at least twice a day. This will also improve wellbeing because of exposure to real daylight (not fake daylight in the form of white fluorescent tubes).

4. Set up your workstation so that you can alternate between sitting and standing.
5. Use an exercise ball to sit on instead of an office chair. This uses your core muscles to stay upright. But beware the rolling ball in terms of office injuries and be sure to get the right size ball for your height.
6. Create a set of stretching exercises to do every hour away from your desk. This will help your muscles and rest your eyes.
7. Improve your core muscles through activities outside of work. pilates, yoga, martial arts etc., are great to improve your core muscles, which in turn will help when sitting for prolonged hours.
8. Set workable hours. It's all about balance. Where possible, try not to sit at a computer for more than six hours per day without significant breaks. Get good amounts of sleep rather than working all hours of the day and night.

It seems basic to make these suggestions but no doubt you don't do enough activity during the day. There are always deadlines to keep or your novel is really going well. Time gets away from you and at the end of the day you realise that you've chained yourself to the desk and have a headache. If you have to set a timer to remind yourself, do it!

Beware the Writers Diet

It's amazing how much fuel you need to make your brain function well. You would think that because you aren't moving much, that you could go all day without food. But we still need our body to function well, and keep our immunity at its peak. The problem with many writers (or office workers) is that they eat lots of snacks and drink copious amounts of tea and coffee, even alcohol. This can be because of boredom, procrastination, laziness or plain mindlessness.

To look after your body, you need to become mindful. If you're feeling sluggish, don't reach for your sixth Tim Tam. You most likely need some fresh air and to get moving, not more sugar.

Getting up to make a cup of tea is good for you in terms of the break and quite often that's why we do it. Our mind is numb, we need caffeine and sugar. The act of getting up to do this is great but maybe this can be replaced every now and again with something else, like a drink of water? Here are some things to think about when it comes to fuelling your body:

1. Limit tea or coffee.
2. Drink as much water as possible (eight glasses is recommended).
3. Limit how many biscuits you eat in a day.
4. Set times to eat during the day that are real meal times and not just enough time to scoff down your food mindlessly.
5. Don't eat at your desk.

6. Don't eat huge, greasy meals that will make you feel queasy and tired for the rest of the day.

7. Eat food that gives you slow release energy for a long time (low GI).

8. Make meals an event where you eat mindfully and feel like you have had a break.

There's no way around it. If you write, you need to sit in front of a screen and type on a keyboard. Maybe in the future there'll be some better invention but I can't imagine what that might be. Anything that requires us to sit and formulate our thoughts into words requires us to sit at a desk. Even if we dictate it into a voice memo and have our computer convert it to words, we still need to go into that document and make it coherent. Writing and any kind of data entry require long periods of time sitting or standing in one position. This puts pressure on our body.

No matter what activity we put our body through, we will decline with age. Some activities will be worse than others over years of repetition. It always comes back to listening to your body and adjusting it as needed. No one thing will fix it; using your logic and using your body as it was designed to do will keep it at its best. Unfortunately, our body wasn't designed to sit and write all day so the best we can do is look after it and be kind to it.

We all send our car to the mechanic for a tune up, don't we? If not, the car will eventually break down and cost a lot more than if it were serviced regularly. Our body is much, much more important than a car. A car can be replaced easily and while some of our body parts can also be replaced, it's not ideal to treat it that way. In fact, a car may only last about 15 years before it starts having major problems like the need for a new engine. Our body can potentially last 100 years. Treat it with respect and gratitude. Move it, eat well and pamper it. A regular massage won't go astray either. It will relax your muscles, move the blood and lymph around your body, de-stress you and feel great! Think of it as part of your maintenance and you might just keep tapping away at that computer until you're 100.

Biographies

Jonathan Chang has been practicing dentistry since 2009. Of Malaysian-Chinese heritage, he was born and raised in Brisbane, where he attended the Anglican Church Grammar School. Following secondary school, he was part of the foundation year of the Griffith University School of Dentistry, graduating in 2008. He has worked in private practices between the Gold Coast and Brisbane, with an interest in endodontics and comestic dentistry.

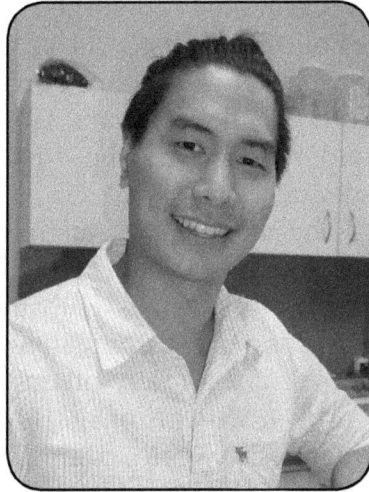

Between 2014 and 2016, Jonathan decided to take a career break to backpack around the world. His travels took him to some amazing places in over 80 countries across 7 continents. His favourite destinations were Antarctica, the Galapagos and Iceland. In his spare time, Jonathan enjoys cooking, learning new languages, watching cricket and rugby, and of course planning his next vacation.

Jonathan believes the importance of dentistry goes far beyond basic oral hygiene, as the mouth acts as a 'window' to the rest of the body and one's general health and wellbeing at every stage of life.

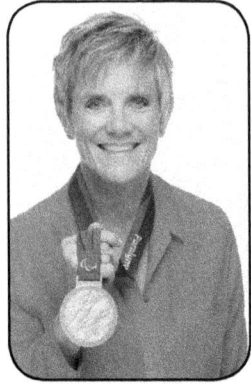

Carol Cooke AM was born in Canada and worked as a Police Officer for 14 years on the Toronto Police Force. Four of those years were undercover in the drug squad.

She moved to Australia for love and had her life thrown into chaos with the diagnosis of a chronic illness. Undeterred, she set herself goals many others wouldn't have dared. Carol, at 55 years of age, is the oldest female Trike rider in the world, competing internationally and has three Paralympic gold medals to her credit as well as five World Championships. She continues to set goals most half her age wouldn't and says that she will continue to challenge herself until the day she is put in a pine box!

Carol believes that anyone can overcome adversity, accept change and find hidden courage and their own gold within themselves.

She truly believes that if you dare to face your fears and believe in yourself you can overcome anything.

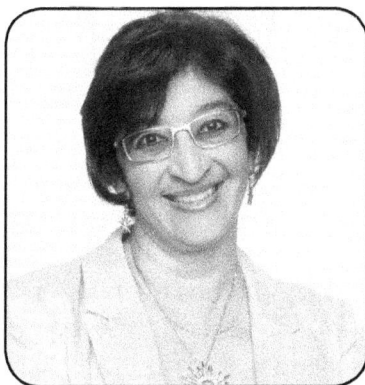

Vanita Dahia is a pharmacist, naturopath, clinical and Mental Health nutritionist, Ayurvedic consultant and Fellow in Anti-ageing and Regenerative Medicine.

Working as a clinical consultant for a functional pathology laboratory, she provides technical assistance to doctors, naturopaths, pharmacists and Allied Health practitioners internationally. Offering extensive experience as a pharmacist in conventional and integrative medicine, she has worked in community and hospital pharmacies as well as the pharmaceutical industry in South Africa and Australia. She owned and managed one of the oldest traditional compounding pharmacies in Australia for 20 years. Vanita has a wealth of information on bio-identical hormone replacement therapy, alternative cancer therapies, custom tailored nutritional medicine and cosmaceutical skin therapy. She continues to update her expertise with current concepts in Biomedical Balance and Integrative Medicine.

Valuing the principle of optimal integrative health to empower, heal, and serve, Vanita incorporates her pharmaceutical compounding knowledge together with herbalism, homoeopathy, ayurvedic medicine and energy medicine to assist others in achieving the best health outcomes.

Vanita is a passionate specialist in the fields of science based nutritional and environmental medicine, and has a special interest in chronic complex conditions such as CFS, FM, IBS, Menopause, Andropause, adrenal fatigue, and mental health such as anxiety and depression.

Nikki Elis has been a personal trainer since 1992 and a sessional academic in the College of Exercise and Sport Science at Victoria University since 2000. Nikki is a passionate advocate for exercise, and in particular women lifting weights. Nikki runs an award winning personal training studio in Macleod in Melbourne's North East and in her private life is happily married to Andrew and spends many hours with their kids Fraser and Sophie at the local pony clubs, soccer clubs and BMX tracks.

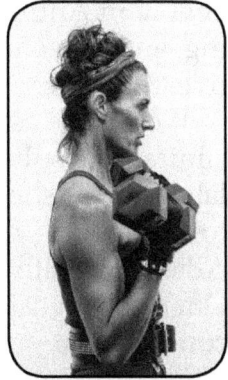

With her own family history of chronic disease and in her 40s herself, **Deborah Harrison** realised she wanted to help other men and women achieve the ultimate combination of lifestyle balance so that

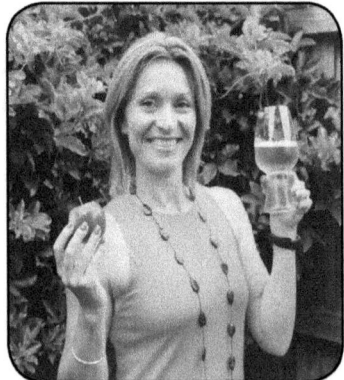

all men and women over 40 could live the life they desire. Using her years of experience as a Nutritionist, Personal Trainer and pilates instructor, Deborah created her own 7 part health & lifestyle program called 'Drink Beer Be Healthy' that teaches men and women all they need to know to make sure that they can achieve everything they want and with a work-life balance. Deborah is a highly sought-after educator conducting seminars and talks around lifestyle changes at private businesses as well as councils and other public companies. Deborah also presents programs for Diabetes Australia where she teaches a government funded educational program to help over 45s make changes in their lives. With all of her experience, Deborah is passionate about helping as many men and women as she can. Through education, she hopes to reduce the rates of health related diseases as well as allowing people to live full and healthy lives.

After completing a Bachelor Degree in Science (majoring in chemistry and biochemistry) at Sydney University, **Kylie Hennessy** began teaching yoga. Kylie practiced intensely in various forms of yoga such as Okido Yoga, Ki Yoga, and Astanga Yoga while completing a four-

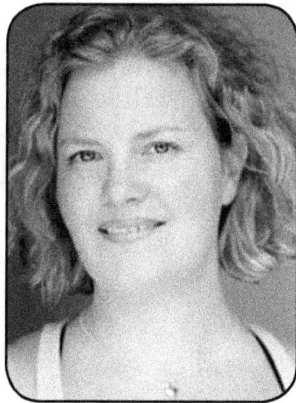

year apprenticeship style of training with Body Mind Unlimited in Sydney to teach Hatha Yoga.

From then her life was all about yoga, meditation and healing modalities. Over many years, Kylie explored the chakra system and energy reading – in particular the amazing healing qualities of the heart chakra with Karima Hinterleitner, long-term follower of the enlightened Mystic Osho. Kylie worked closely and trained with Traditional Chinese Medicine Practitioner and tai chi and Qi Gong teacher Angela Zhu, and trained with Japanese Yoga teachers such as Peter Masters of Zen Central and Jack Marshall of Zen Renaissance Centre. She has studied with many of Australia's leading yoga therapists such as Leigh Blashki, Annette Loudon, Sal Flynn and Liz Bennett. She enjoys the work of scientists such as Dr Candice Pert, Dr Bruce Lipton and Dr Jo Dispenza, whose work compliments her own knowledge and experience of yoga.

The sum of this experience has recently expanded into running three yoga studios and Natural Health Clinics across Sydney and at the Sydney Pregnancy Centre. The centre warmly welcomes all kinds of people to enjoy a range of yoga classes, yoga therapy and other mind-body therapies offering a place of healing, community, sanctuary and support.

Anthony Kilner is a psychic medium, multi-published author, education-al facilitator, men-tor, energy work-er, freelance photo journalist, speaker and musician. He is also qualified in trance healing, massage and is a reiki and seichim master.

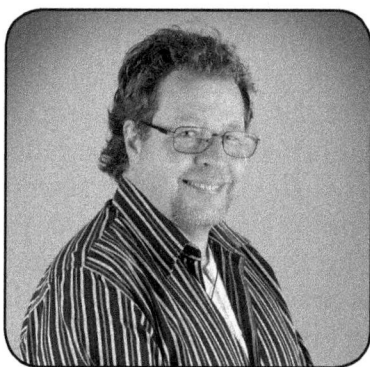

Having studied Vibrational Healing and meditation techniques in India and Australia, Anthony has come to respect them as a powerful tools to promote ongoing wellbeing as it works on the entire physical body, encouraging self-healing.

After actively working with Spirit for over ten years as a Psychic Medium at various locations, Anthony has now created a beautiful working and teaching environment in Research Victoria where he operates his businesses – Bridging Realms – www.bridgingrealms.com.au, Ant e Fiction and The Spiritual Coach.

Anthony is passionate about assisting people with a holistic approach to living and working and how to find the right work/life balance. In 2013 he started his newest business, The Spiritual Coach, and also wrote his first book, *Secret Spiritual Business – Unlocking the Power to Holistic Success,* where he shares a plethora of knowledge and personal experiences on how to achieve success while doing what you love and working from home.

Anthony launched the first in a trilogy of co-authored books, *Healthy Mind* in 2015, with *Healthy Body* following in 2017. He has also launched a new book called *Practical Mediumship – A Guide to Understanding Psychics, Mediums, Dreams and Physical and Metaphysical Information.* The world of Subjective and Objective information is covered in more detail than has been discussed in his chapter on the Metaphysical World.

Mary Jo Mc Veigh is a trained trauma therapist and an accredited mental health social worker. She has a passion for exploring and studying comprehensive bodies of knowledge, bringing this emphasis for diversity of wisdom to her work, creatively utilising it within her therapeutic and leadership practice. Mary Jo completed her Honours degree in Social Science in 1983 and worked in the community of North Belfast in the United Kingdom, before returning to university and completing a Masters degree in Social Work in 1986. She has been working with vulnerable persons both within Australia and internationally since then, and is the CEO and founder of both Cara House and CaraCare.

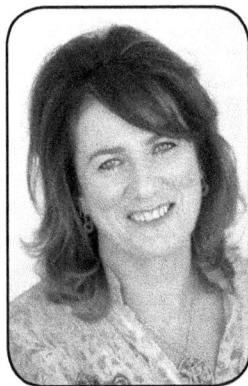

Mary Jo is acknowledged in her field as an expert in child protection, trauma therapy and leadership coaching. Mary Jo's expertise has been sought on advisory panels such as the NSW Domestic Violence reforms and the Royal Commission into institutional abuse. She has also presented at national and international conferences.

Mary Jo's work has been published in professional journals. She has also written numerous training programs for practitioners and managers in government and charitable organisations within Australia. Mary Jo has published three innovative social work resources for working therapeutically with children and young people. The most beloved one, Wrapped in Angels, has received praise nationally and internationally. Mary Jo is currently working on other exciting works, so keep an eye out.

A former journalist, **Julie O'Connell Seamer** writes for health magazines, supplement brands and well-being websites. She has also practiced as a Naturopath for almost 20 years – in community health centres, private clinics, and city to rural wellness outlets Australia-wide, focusing on women's hormones, sports nutrition, anti-ageing, food intolerances and 'mystery illnesses'.

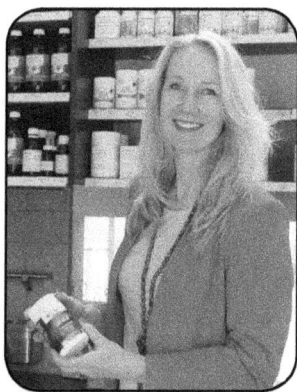

Julie survived her partner's suicide while she was pregnant with their son. This tragedy (culminated by his chronic health issues) crystalised a knowing she'd long suspected – sickness is the body's message system of alerting us to certain imbalances that need our attention. It could be a short attack of the common cold, on-going discomfort from a lingering condition or a potentially life-threatening disease that's presented in your life. According to Julie, these circumstances can cultivate insights into the deeper recesses of ourselves and offer a chance to draw on our true grit. She is passionate in supporting her patients in their mental health needs and in reducing the stigma of depression in our society. Her upcoming book, 'Your Body is Your Teacher', is a compilation of 'light bulb' moments from personal experiences and real cases. Julie currently practices at Renew Clinic in Macleod, Victoria.

Blaise van Hecke is co-owner and Publisher at Busybird Publishing. She is also a writer, photographer and artist. She has been published in the short story anthology, *Mud Puddles* (May 08), *Blue Crow Magazine*, *[untitled]* issue two, came second in the bi-annual short story competition with the Society of Women Writers of Victoria 2007 for her story 'The Eleventh Summer', and is the author of *The Book Book: 12 steps to successful publishing*, as well as *Who is*

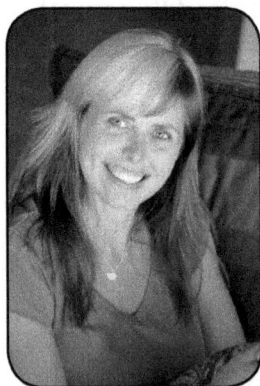

a Cheeky Monkey? Her photographs have been used for book covers, CD covers and promotional literature.

Blaise enjoys writing and travelling and hopes to publish a book that combines both. She runs various workshops for Busybird about writing, editing, and publishing, and is popularly in demand for talks about publishing in general.

What Blaise loves most is nurturing an author through the self-publishing process, and the look on their face when they finally have their book in their hands.

Find out more about Blaise at www. thebookchick.com.au.

Megan Wright IAT, was born in Somerset, England before migrating with her family to Melbourne, Australia. Her passion for the hair and beauty industry began with an inpromtu haircut on her two year old brother when she was at the tender age of four, and she has never looked back.

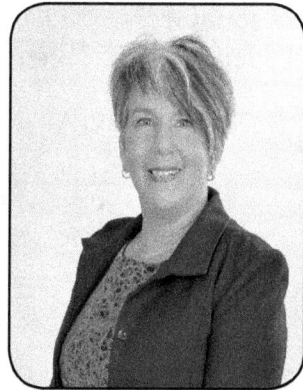

Megan has owned and managed award-winning hairdressing salons in Melbourne and regional Victoria and trained several award-winning apprentices before branching out as a leading educator for Victoria University, Ballarat University, Pivot Point College, and, currently at Federation University.

Now with thirty years of experience in the Hair and Beauty Industry, Megan is highly sought after as a speaker, trainer and business mentor. Megan has published her internationally recognised business book, *Your Salon Success, 12 Step Blueprint to Profit Potential,* and is currently one of only a few Clinical Trichologists in Australia.

As a Trichologist, hair and scalp specialist, Megan sees many patients who are suffering with hair loss and other hair and scalp conditions. She has a practice in Ballarat where she services patients from all around Regional Victoria.

Megan's passion is the education and empowerment of individuals to create better opportunities in all aspects of their business and personal lives.

Her motto is: 'Energise, Empower, Evolve!'

Title: *Healthy Mind*

Price: $25.00

Publication Date: 23 October 2015

Format: Paperback (210x135mm, 182 pages)

ISBN: 978 1 925260 78 8

Category: Nonfiction

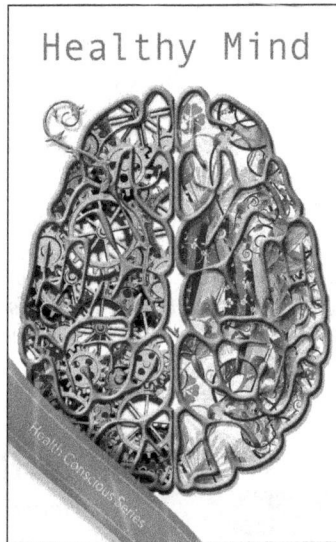

How do you keep a healthy mind?

In the hustle and bustle of our everyday lives, it's a question that's often neglected. We may diet or exercise to take care of our bodies, but little thought is given to good mental health. Mental health issues – things like depression, anxiety, etc. – are on the rise. A general malaise of constant tiredness, agitation, or even anger, is common.

How do you feel? As you read this blurb, pause a moment and reflect on your mental health. Is your outlook positive, constructive, and purposeful? Or do you find yourself often flustered, uptight, and confused? Unfortunately, we can run with these patterns so long they become our mindset. But surely you want something better. Surely you deserve something better?

Healthy Mind features articles from ten diverse professionals who explore the concept of a healthy mind from their specific viewpoint, and offer tips and exercises on creating and maintaining good mental health.

Simple, interesting, and compelling, *Healthy Mind* has something for everybody, and is sure to become an invaluable guide.

Joffa: Isn't That Life?

Price: $25.00
Author: Jeff 'Joffa' Corfe
Publication Date: June 2015
Format: Softcover (234x153mm, 205 pages)
ISBN: 978 1 925260 29 8
Category: Autobiography

Everybody believes Joffa's a loud-mouthed bogan from the Collingwood Football Club Cheer Squad. But learn about his teenage homelessness, his tireless charity work, and what he thinks about supporting Collingwood.

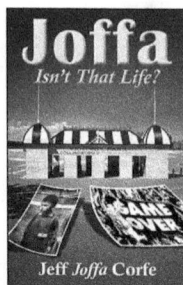

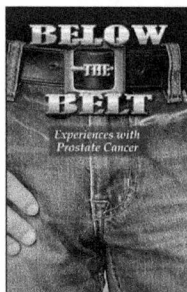

Below the Belt

Experiences with Prostate Cancer
Author: Various
Price: $25.00
Publication Date: November 2014
Format: Paperback (234x153mm, 205 pages)
ISBN: 978 0 9925547 3 6
Category: Nonfiction

Everyday people talk about their experiences with prostate cancer, their treatments, the trials they've faced, and what they've learned.

Journey

Experiences with Breast Cancer
Author: Various
Price: $25.00
Publication Date: February 2012
Format: Paperback (234x153mm, 326 pages)
ISBN: 978 0 987153 80 7
Category: Nonfiction

Take a journey with everyday people as they share their experiences with breast cancer. Their stories and poetry offer insights into every facet of their travails.

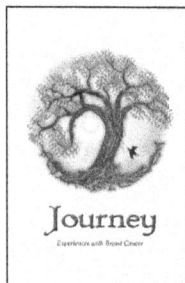

The Book Book
12 Steps to Successful Publishing
Author: Blaise van Hecke
Price: $15.00
Publication Date: February 2014
Format: Paperback (181x111mm, 148 pages)
ISBN: 978 0 992432 50 8
Category: Nonfiction

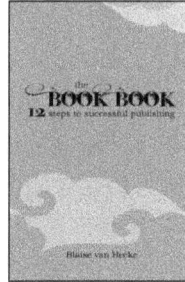

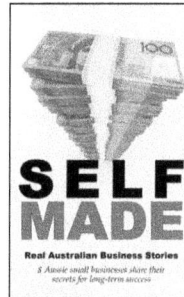

Everyone has a book in them, but where do we start? The Book Book *breaks the process into manageable steps, providing tips, insider knowledge, and the inspiration to get your book published!*

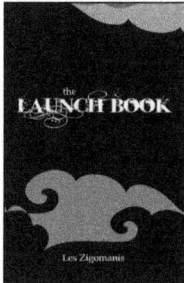

The Launch Book
The Little Guide to Launching Your Book
Author: Les Zigomanis
Price: $12.00
Publication Date: April 2015
Format: Paperback (181x111mm, 70 pages)
ISBN: 978 0 99243250 8
Category: Nonfiction

You've written a book but don't know what to do next. This simple and fun guide will show you how to have a great launch and celebrate your book coming into the world.

Self Made
Real Australian Business Stories
Author: Various
Price: $15.00
Publication Date: February 2014
Format: Paperback (111x181mm, 143 pages)
ISBN: 978 0 992487 43 0
Category: Nonfiction

Eight biopics from business owners who've been there and done that. If you're looking for hints and tips in business, don't go any further!

Busybird Publishing is a boutique micro-publisher based in the heart of Montmorency, Victoria.

We publish a handful of titles yearly, trying to combine quality and entertainment with some altruistic outcome, e.g. raising awareness for a particular condition (as our glorious coffee table photography book, *Walk With Me* – a journal of Kev Howlett's trek up to Mount Everest Base Camp and back – raised awareness of Charcot-Marie-Tooth disease), and/or donate a portion of proceeds for books to various foundations (such as Women Helping Women, Breast Cancer Victoria, the Prostate Cancer Foundation, the Epilepsy Foundation, Vision Australia, the Indigenous Literacy Foundation), and with this book to the Go for Gold Scholarship.

We also run workshops on various forms of writing (fiction, nonfiction, memoir), publishing, and photography, and an annual two-day writing retreat; host a monthly Open Mic Night (the third Wednesday of every month); and hold competitions to help aspiring writers get published or win mentoring.

To learn more about Busybird Publishing, check out our website at **www.busybird.com.au**.

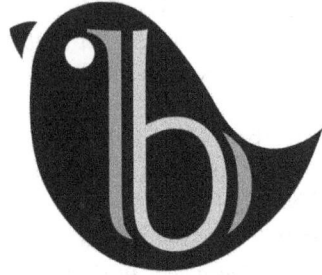